AUDREY LATSHAW SUTTON, R.N.

Case Reviewer, Hospital Division of
Blue Cross of Philadelphia;
Nursing Consultant, James Associates
Medical Advisors, Swarthmore, Pa.
Formerly Clinical Instructor of Practical Nursing,
Wilmington General Hospital, Wilmington, Delaware;
Instructor of Practical Nursing,
H. Fletcher Brown Vocational School, Wilmington;
Member, Committee for the Development
of Instructional Materials,
Practical Nurse Program of the Wilmington
Public Schools, Wilmington;
Director of Nursing Service,
Edgewood General Hospital, Berlin, New Jersey.

THIRD EDITION

WORKBOOK FOR PRACTICAL NURSES

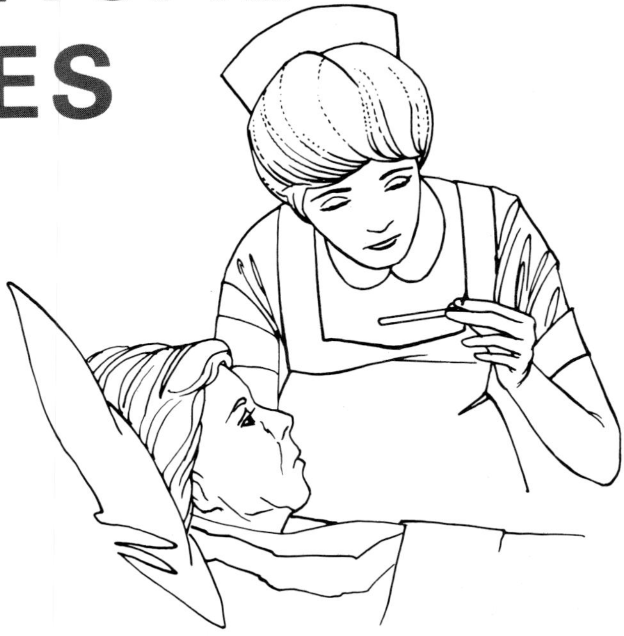

. SAUNDERS COMPANY Philadelphia London Toronto 1969

W. B. Saunders Company: West Washington Square
Philadelphia, Pa. 19105

12 Dyott Street
London W. C. 1

1835 Yonge Street
Toronto, Ontario 295

Workbook for Practical Nurses

PREFACE

Once again a revision of this workbook has been found desirable in order to keep pace with the current trends in practical nursing. The cordial reception accorded the second edition has indicated that few major changes have been needed, but numerous minor improvements have been made. Among them are the addition of new drawings and some rearrangement of topics. An example of the latter is the shifting of the material on the male genitourinary system to a new chapter on the reproductive system that combines both male and female components.

All references to textbooks have been brought carefully up to date. An innovation intended to add both interest and currency is the inclusion in this edition of references to articles in the periodical literature of practical nursing.

The functions of the book remain the same. The book is keyed for use with all the current practical nurse textbooks. The author suggests that several of the references and a portion of the problems in each chapter be assigned to the student for preclass preparation. There are situation problems which may be used for classroom discussion and laboratory periods. Additional assignments which are suitable for home study or testing materials are included. The entire book is designed to simplify learning processes while emphasizing those topics which are of particular importance to the practical nurse. The book encompasses all areas recommended in a curriculum for practical nurse education and may serve as a curriculum guide for the instructor.

The attempt has been made to present the material at a level suitable for both the high school and the adult student. Parts I through IV are intended for use in the preclinical or preparatory program. Parts V through X are intended for use in the clinical program. Each part is assembled in a manner which permits each chapter or chapter subdivision to be utilized as a separate and complete lesson to allow for flexibility in subject presentation. The core approach is used in presenting all subject matter related to disease conditions. Accompanying the common abnormalities of each body system is an anatomy and physiology review and a discussion of diagnostic procedures, medical and surgical treatment, and general nursing care. Diet and drug therapy are included as a part of the medical treatment.

The author is deeply grateful to all those instructors who have reviewed the previous edition of the workbook and have offered extremely helpful suggestions.

Audrey Latshaw Sutton

CONTENTS

PART I

AN ORIENTATION TO NURSING

Chapter 1

HOW PRACTICAL NURSING BEGAN

HISTORY
RECENT TRENDS

REFERENCES

Bush, C. H.: Personal and Vocational Relationships for Practical Nurses. 2nd ed. Philadelphia, W. B. Saunders Co., 1966, Chapters 1 and 5.

Culver, V.: Modern Bedside Nursing. 7th ed. Philadelphia, W. B. Saunders Co., 1969, Chapter 2.

Hoffman, C. P., Lipkin, G. B., and Thompson, E. M.: Simplified Nursing. 8th ed. Philadelphia, J. B. Lippincott Co., 1968, Chapter 1.

Johnston, D. F.: History and Trends of Practical Nursing. St. Louis, The C. V. Mosby Co., 1966, Chapters 1-4.

Rapier, D. K., et al.: Practical Nursing. 3rd ed. St. Louis, The C. V. Mosby Co., Chapter 1.

Rasmussen, S.: Foundations of Practical and Vocational Nursing. New York, The Macmillan Co., 1967, Chapter 1.

Ross, C. F.: Personal and Vocational Relationships in Practical Nursing. 2nd ed. Philadelphia, J. B. Lippincott Co., 1965, Chapter 2.

Stevens, M. K.: Personal and Vocational Relationships of the Practical Nurse. Philadelphia, W. B. Saunders Co., 1967, Chapter 20.

Thompson, E., and Murphy, C.: Textbook of Basic Nursing. Philadelphia, J. B. Lippincott Co., 1966, Chapter 1.

---

1. Who was the first practical nurse?

2. The following persons or groups contributed to the development of nursing as a profession and to the organization of practical nurse training and education. Discuss the role that each played in this field.

A. Florence Nightingale established the first modern school for nurses at St Thomas Hospital in England.

B. Lucinda Ballard established a school of nursing in 1893 for practical nurses. A three month course to train women to give simple nursing care

C. Clara Barton

D. Linda Richards

E. Sisters of Charity

F. Young Women's Christian Association, Central Branch, New York

G. Mr. Thomas Thompson founded the 2nd school for practical nurses in Vermont 1917

H. Household Nursing Association, Boston, Massachusetts - 1918

3. Many advancements have been made in practical nursing recently. The important results of recent accomplishments are:

A. Approved Schools

(1) What is meant by an approved school? In an approved school all admission requirements curriculum standards must meet certain standards. These schools must also have qualified teachers, provide the student with hospital experience and a certain # of hours of instruction

(2) List several advantages of attending an approved school.
A better grade of education
A better opportunity for employment

B. Licensure

(1) How does a practical nurse receive her license?
By completing the required course of study in class and clinic and by taking and successfully passing the state board exam of the state in which she wishes to practice

(2) Why is it important for a practical nurse to be licensed?

(3) In your state, what letters does the licensed practical nurse use after her name? L.V.N. Licensed Vocational nurse

(4) Define the following terms:

(a) Mandatory licensure: a practical nurse may not practice her vocation under this law without a current license.

(b) Permissive licensure: a practical nurse may under this law, practice her vocation providing she does not use the title L.P.N., L.V.N or otherwise represent herself as licensed.

(c) License by waiver a system used for a while after state licensing laws were passed. A practical nurse that was practicing before the law could obtain her license without taking an exam by supplying forms, fee and references of various people.

C. <u>Practical nurse organizations</u>

(1) Briefly discuss the purpose and functions of the nursing organizations to which a practical nurse may belong.

(a) State Association for Practical Nurses

(b) The National Federation of Licensed Practical Nurses

(c) The National Association for Practical Nurse Education and Service

(d) National League for Nursing

(2) List two reasons why it is important for the practical nurse to support these organizations.

(3) Explain how you can become a member of each of the organizations.

Chapter 2

WHAT IS THE PRACTICAL NURSE?

DEFINITION
EDUCATION
DUTIES
FUNCTIONS

REFERENCES

Bush, C. H.: Personal and Vocational Relationships for Practical Nurses, Chapters 2, 3 and 9.
Culver, V.: Modern Bedside Nursing, Chapter 2.
Hoffman, C. P., Lipkin, G., and Thompson, E.: Simplified Nursing, Chapter 1.
Johnston, D.: History and Trends of Practical Nursing, Chapters 5-7.
Morison, L. J., and Farris, M. A.: Approaches for Co-workers in Professional Nursing, Part III, Unit 3.
Rapier, D. K., et al.: Practical Nursing, Chapter 3.
Rasmussen, S.: Foundations of Practical and Vocational Nursing, Chapter.1.
Ross, C. F.: Personal and Vocational Relationships in Practical Nursing, Chapters 1 and 3.
Stevens, M. K.: Personal and Vocational Relationships of the Practical Nurse, Chapters 21 and 22.
Thompson, E., and Murphy, C.: Textbook of Basic Nursing, Chapter 1.

1. What is a practical nurse?

2. List the duties of a practical nurse.

3. What are the requirements for entrance to your school of practical nursing?

4. What is the importance of clinical training as part of the education of practical nurses?

5. Name three good study habits.

6. List five important points to remember when taking notes.

7. Each year more opportunities are being made available to practical nurses. In your community, what positions are available to the practical nurse?

8. Discuss the role of each of the following members of the "health team":

A. Professional nurse

B. Dietitian

C. Orderly

D. Social service worker

E. Physiotherapist

Chapter 3

PROFESSIONAL CONDUCT

PERSONALITY
ETHICS

REFERENCES

Bush, C. H.: Personal and Vocational Relationships for Practical Nurses, Chapters 3 and 4.
Culver, V.: Modern Bedside Nursing, Chapters 3 and 5.
Gill, H. Z.: Basic Nursing, Chapter 2.
Hoffman, C. P., Lipkin, G., and Thompson, E.: Simplified Nursing, Chapters 2 and 4.
Rapier, D. K., et al.: Practical Nursing, Chapter 4.
Rasmussen, S.: Foundations of Practical and Vocational Nursing, Chapter 1.
Ross, C. F.: Personal and Vocational Relationships in Practical Nursing, Chapters 4 and 5.
Stevens, M. K.: Personal and Vocational Relationships of the Practical Nurse, Units 1 to 3.
Thompson, E., and Murphy, C.: Textbook of Basic Nursing, Chapter 3.

---

1. In your own words, define maturity.

2. Name the three personality traits which you think are the most important for a nurse to possess. Tell the reasons why you have chosen each of these.

3. List three important rules of etiquette for the nurse in her relationships with

   A. The patient

   B. Her co-workers

   C. Her superiors

4. Name several habits which are important in preventing the nurse from becoming emotionally tense and worrisome:

5. What approach would you use in handling the following?

A. Your head nurse asks you to give an enema. You have never been taught how to give an enema.

B. You are assigned to the care of a patient in a semi-private room. Another patient in the room, who is someone else's assignment, asks for a bedpan.

C. You observe that while on duty Miss A., a graduate nurse, is doing many things that are not considered to be good ethical conduct.

D. It is time for your coffee break, but things are hectic, and you don't see how you can manage to get away.

E. In a loud voice your head nurse criticizes your work in front of everyone.

F. Miss D., a patient, wants to know your confidential opinion of her doctor.

6. Make a list of "Do's" and "Don'ts" applying to a nurse's appearance when on duty.

Do's	Don'ts

Chapter 4

LEGAL OBLIGATIONS

REFERENCES

Bush, C. H.: Personal and Vocational Relationships for Practical Nurses, Chapter 11.
Creighton, M.: Law Every Nurse Should Know. Philadelphia, W. B. Saunders Co., 1957.
Culver, V.: Modern Bedside Nursing, Chapter 4.
Hoffman, C. P., Lipkin, G., and Thompson, E.: Simplified Nursing, Chapter 5.
Rapier, D. K., et al.: Practical Nursing, p. 595.
Rasmussen, S.: Foundations of Practical and Vocational Nursing, Chapter 50.
Ross, C. F.: Personal and Vocational Relationships in Practical Nursing, Chapter 7.
Stevens, M. K.: Personal and Vocational Relationships of the Practical Nurse, Chapter 26.
Thompson, E., and Murphy, C.: Textbook of Basic Nursing, Chapter 54.

1. Match the following legal terms with their definitions.

3 a.	Slander	1.	Deliberate commission or omission of an act forbidden by law.
1 b.	Crime	2.	Threat by the nurse in which the patient is in fear of harmful conduct.
5 c.	Libel	3.	Untrue damaging verbal statement
4 d.	Negligence	4.	Not doing what is normally expected in practical nursing
2 e.	Assault	5.	Untrue and damaging written statement

2. What conditions are necessary to make a will valid in your state?

3. Each nurse has legal responsibilities in the performance of her duties and in carrying out orders given by the physician. Be prepared to discuss each of the following situations concerning a type of legal obligation to the nursing profession.

A. Practical Nurse E. has promised Dr. Jones that she will care for his patient beginning Friday morning. In the meantime Practical Nurse E. decides to accompany a friend to a resort on Friday and asks you to care for the patient. What will you do?

B. Mrs. B., an ambulatory patient, is to have a hot water bottle applied to her abdomen. You are busy and ask her to fill the hot water bottle herself. She does so, but the water is too warm and she is burned. Who is responsible for this accident? Why?

C. Dr. Black and Dr. Jones each have a patient with a skin allergy on the ward on which you are on duty. Dr. Black has ordered cornstarch baths for his patient, who is progressing well. Dr. Jones has not ordered this treatment for his patient, and the patient apparently is not improving. Should you, as the nurse, conclude that Dr. Jones is negligent? Why?

4. Place a check mark in front of the nursing acts which require a doctor's order.

✓ A. Giving an enema
✓ B. Giving a glass of water
✓ C. Rubbing a back
___ D. Giving an aspirin
✓ E. Massaging the legs
✓ F. Taking the temperature
___ G. Giving a hot water bottle
___ H. Elevating the head of the bed
✓ I. Elevating the foot of the bed
✓ J. Combing hair

PART II

UNDERSTANDING HEALTH AND SOCIETY

Chapter 5

PERSONAL HEALTH

PHYSICAL AND MENTAL HEALTH
HEALTH TEACHING

REFERENCES

Culver, V.: Modern Bedside Nursing, Chapter 22.
Hasler, D.: Personal, Home and Community Health. New York, The Macmillan Co., 1967.
Hoffman, C. P., Lipkin, G., and Thompson, E.: Simplified Nursing, pp. 16-18, 29-41.
Rapier, D. K., et al.: Practical Nursing, Chapter 2.
Rasmussen, S.: Foundations of Practical and Vocational Nursing, Chapter 2.
Thompson, E., and Murphy, C.: Textbook of Basic Nursing, Chapters 4 and 5.

JOURNALS

Block, Marvin A.: Understanding alcoholism. J. Practical Nursing, 16:27, Nov. 1966.
Young, Lieselotte Doerr: Understanding the alcoholic. J. Practical Nursing, 18:20, Nov. 1968.

---

1. Define health.

2. Discuss ways in which a nurse can develop good health habits under the following:

   A. Posture

   B. Care of feet

   C. Eating habits

   D. Care of skin

   E. Care of hair

3. How can a practical nurse be a health teacher?

4. Discuss the hazards involved when a nurse allows herself to become consistently overfatigued.

5. True or False. Place a T in front of the statements that are true and an F in front of the statements that are false.

T 1. Alcoholism is an illness.
F 2. An optometrist is a physician with specialized training in all types of eye diseases.
F 3. People as a whole are beginning to understand that sexual relations and emotions have no definite connections.
F 4. Shower or bathtub bathing is harmful during menstruation.
T 5. An exodontist is a specialist in tooth extraction.
T 6. If you have a cold, you are responsible for protecting other people.
F 7. To keep mentally healthy, one should have little or no flexibility in emotions.
T 8. A chiropodist is a specialist in all types of foot disorders.
F 9. Normal bowel elimination includes having a bowel movement at least once or twice daily.
F 10. Reading in bed is harmful to the eyes.

Chapter 6

COMMUNITY HEALTH

HISTORY OF PUBLIC HEALTH
PUBLIC HEALTH SERVICES

REFERENCES

Culver, V.: Modern Bedside Nursing, Chapter 24.
Hasler, D.: Personal, Home and Community Health.
Hoffman, C. P., Lipkin, G., and Thompson, E.: Simplified Nursing, pp. 18-29.
Rapier, D. K., et al.: Practical Nursing, Chapter 7.
Rasmussen, S.: Foundations of Practical and Vocational Nursing, pp. 41-53.
Thompson, E., and Murphy, C.: Textbook of Basic Nursing, Chapter 6.
U. S. Department of Health, Education, and Welfare: Brief Explanation of Functions.

---

1. Briefly describe your understanding of the term "public health."

2. During which century were most of the public health agencies organized?

3. Public health organizations are of two types: (1) Official, or governmental, those agencies which are financed by the tax dollars of citizens; (2) Nonofficial, or voluntary, those agencies financed by voluntary contributions. Official health agencies may be national, state or local. The majority of the national health agencies concerned with community health are divisions of the U.S. Department of Health, Education, and Welfare. This agency cooperates with the states in fulfilling its functions. The following is a list of the five major units of the U.S. Department of Health, Education, and Welfare. What are the major services of each of these units?

   A. Public Health Service

B. Social Security Administration

C. Food and Drug Administration

D. Office of Education

E. Office of Vocational Rehabilitation

4. List the major nonofficial, or voluntary, health agencies in your community and give the location and functions of each.

5. When and where was the World Health Organization formed? What are its functions?

6. Who is the present Surgeon General of the United States Public Health Service?

7. What is the difference between the "visiting nurse" and the "public health nurse"?

8. Where is your local health department located?

9. What regulations can your local health department enforce?

10. What is the location of the principal office of your state health department?

Chapter 7

FAMILY LIFE

FAMILY STRUCTURE AND FUNCTIONS
FACTORS WHICH INFLUENCE THE FAMILY

REFERENCES

Culver, V.: Modern Bedside Nursing, Chapter 23.
Hasler, D.: The Practical Nurse and Today's Family. New York, The Macmillan Co., 1964.
Hoffman, C. P., Lipkin, G., and Thompson, E.: Simplified Nursing, Chapter 6.
Rapier, D. K., et al.: Practical Nursing, Chapter 5.
Rasmussen, S.: Foundations of Practical and Vocational Nursing, pp. 21-24.
Thompson, E., and Murphy, C.: Textbook of Basic Nursing, Chapter 10.

---

1. Define the word "family" as it is known today.

2. Compare family life of the past with that of the present. Discuss the changes that have taken place.

3. What factors should be considered when selecting a marriage partner?

4. List the functions of the modern family.

5. List some factors which may influence family life.

6. Discuss the satisfactory relations which should exist between:

   A. Husband and wife

   B. Parent and child

   C. Brother and sister

7. What are some causes of broken marriages?

8. Discuss how family adjustments may be made in the following possible situations of conflict:

A. Difference in attitudes

B. Coming of children

C. Domineering in-laws

D. Emotional problems

9. Which community agencies are of value in stabilizing family life?

10. Why is it important for the nurse to understand something about family life?

Chapter 8

CHILD GROWTH AND DEVELOPMENT

PHYSICAL GROWTH
MENTAL GROWTH

REFERENCES

Culver, V.: Modern Bedside Nursing, Chapters 17-20.
Hasler, D.: The Practical Nurse and Today's Family, Chapters 2-5, 7-13, 18.
Hoffman, C. P., Lipkin, G., and Thompson, E.: Simplified Nursing, Chapter 7.
Rapier, D. K., et al.: Practical Nursing, pp. 466-473
Rasmussen, S.: Foundations of Practical and Vocational Nursing, pp. 584-641.
Thompson, D.: Pediatrics for Practical Nurses. Philadelphia, W. B. Saunders Co., 1965, Chapters 7, 9, 11, 13, and 15.
Thompson, E., and Murphy, C.: Textbook of Basic Nursing, Chapters 8 and 9.

---

1. Explain the growth process of the child.

2. What are the basic needs of the child?

3. List some ways in which an adult can direct children toward becoming well-adjusted adults.

4. What effect can environment have on a child's growth and development? Give examples.

5. List the personality traits a pediatric nurse should possess.

6. Define heredity.

7. List some characteristics which may be inherited.

8. What are the nutritional needs of the child? How do these needs vary in different stages of childhood?

9. How much sleep does the child need daily? How does the amount vary with age?

10. Discuss the importance of play to the child's life.

11. At what approximate age should the average infant be able to do the following:

A. Grasp objects

B. Sit alone

C. Crawl or creep

D. Stand alone

E. Walk alone

12. At what approximate age could the following be initiated in infant or child care?

A. Placing rattle in hand

B. Propping into sitting position for short periods

C. Allowing to hold bottle

D. Allowing to drink from cup

E. Bladder training

F. Bowel training

G. Providing noise-making play materials

H. Use of walker

I. Providing hard foods, such as bread crusts

J. Concentrating effort on language development

K. Use of tricycle

L. Learning to count

M. Visit to dentist

N. Preparing for physiological changes which occur at puberty

O. Permission to select own clothes

P. Permission to "date"

13. What should be done about the following childhood problems?

A. Bed wetting

B. Thumb sucking

C. Refusal to eat

D. Masturbation

E. Temper tantrums

Chapter 9

THE AGED

SOCIAL AND ECONOMIC ASPECTS
PREPARATION FOR OLD AGE

REFERENCES

Culver, V.: Modern Bedside Nursing, Chapter 50.
Hasler, D.: The Practical Nurse and Today's Family, Chapters 22-28.
Hoffman, C. P., Lipkin, G., and Thompson, E.: Simplified Nursing, p. 354.
Newton, K.: Geriatric Nursing. St. Louis, The C. V. Mosby Co., 1954.
Rapier, D. K., et al.: Practical Nursing, pp. 439-441
Rasmussen, S.: Foundations of Practical and Vocational Nursing, pp. 657-660.
Stevens, M. K.: Geriatric Nursing. Philadelphia, W. B. Saunders Co., 1966, Chapters 2 and 3.
Thompson, E., and Murphy, C.: Textbook of Basic Nursing, pp. 107-110.

---

1. When does a person become old?

2. What physical changes accompany old age?

3. What are the basic needs of the aged?

4. Discuss some of the problems of growing old.

5. How could you, as a nurse, help someone prepare for old age?

6. Why is more emphasis being placed on the older generation each year?

7. Explain how the following can be of assistance to elderly persons:

   A. Social Security Act

   B. Old Age Assistance Program

8. List the organizations in your community which offer assistance to the aged.

9. List opportunities which may be provided to enable aging persons to make useful contributions to the family and to the community.

10. Be prepared to discuss the following situations:

A. Grandmother's recent death left grandfather living in the house by himself. Should the family insist that grandfather sell the house and all his belongings and move in with them? Why?

B. Grandma, who lives with her son Bob and his family, loves to collect all types of calendars. Bob's wife didn't mind it when Grandma hung the calendars on her bedroom walls for display in the old house, but the family recently moved into a new house and Bob's wife doesn't want the walls ruined or cluttered with old calendars. What advice would you offer this family? Why?

C. Mr. and Mrs. Jones were recently faced with a decision of either allowing Grandfather to move in with them or paying for his room and board at a home for the aged. Either alternative was possible as far as living space and finances were concerned. They decided to send Grandfather to the home. What are your opinions of this decision?

D. Your Aunt Ada, who lives in a home for the elderly, comes to visit you occasionally. During these visits she always insists that she will take over the meal preparation and allow you to rest. She proceeds to rummage through the refrigerator and pantry to see what she can cook for dinner. Her menus are not suitable for your family, and her dishes are unappetizing and tasteless. What should be done in this situation? Why?

PART III

STRUCTURE AND FUNCTION OF THE BODY

Chapter 10

THE BODY AS A WHOLE

REFERENCES

Anthony, C. P.: Structure and Function of the Body. 3rd ed. St. Louis, The C. V. Mosby Co., 1968, Chapter 1.
Culver, V., Modern Bedside Nursing, Chapter 6.
Dienhart, C. M.: Basic Human Anatomy and Physiology. Philadelphia, W. B. Saunders Co., 1967, Chapter 1.
Hoffman, C. P., Lipkin, G., and Thompson, E.: Simplified Nursing, Chapter 9.
Manner, H.: Elements of Anatomy and Physiology. Philadelphia, W. B. Saunders Co., 1962, Chapters 1-3.
Memmler, R. L.: The Human Body in Health and Disease. 2nd ed. Philadelphia, J. B. Lippincott Co., 1962, Chapter 1, pp. 32-35.
Rapier, D. K., et al.: Practical Nursing, pp. 39-42.
Rasmussen, S.: Foundations of Practical and Vocational Nursing, Chapter 28.
Thompson, E., and Murphy, C.: Textbook of Basic Nursing, Chapter 11, pp. 125-126.

1. The cell is the basic microscopic unit of all body structures. There are various kinds, but each is composed of cytoplasm, a nucleus and cell membrane. Draw the parts of the cell and label them correctly in Figure 1.

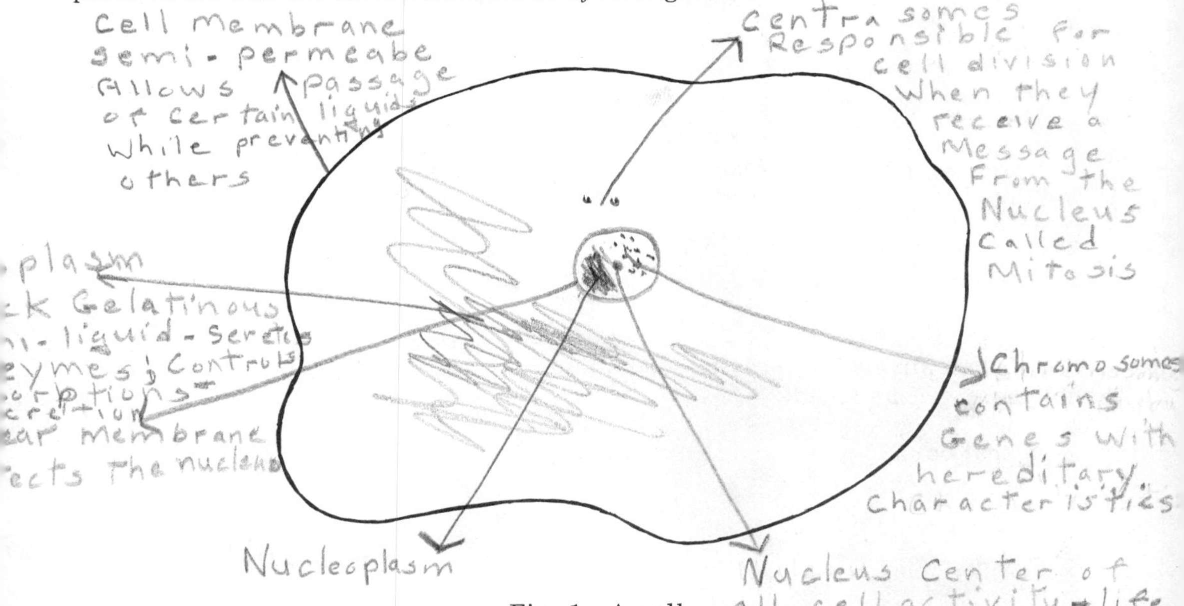

Fig. 1. A cell.

2. A tissue is a group of similar cells performing one special function. What are the functions of each of the following types of tissue?

A. Muscular : provides Movement of cells by contracting

B. Connective : serves as binding, packing or attaching tissue for other organs.

C. Nerve :
Is highly specialized; conducts impulses to and from the brain. It also makes up the cells of the brain.

D. Epithelial tissues serve as Protection

E. Vascular, or liquid Serve as a transportation system, helps combat infection, and helps to neutralize Poisons.

3. A membrane is a thin layer of one or more types of tissue which covers or lines a part of the body for protection.

A. In what parts of the body is each of the following types of membrane located?

(1) Cutaneous : on the skin

(2) Serous : in the abdominal Cavity

(3) Synovial : in the joint Cavities.

(4) Mucous in the Nose ; the respiratory tract

B. Which types of tissue combine to form the cutaneous membrane?

Connective Blood
Epithelial

4. An organ is a group of tissues grouped together to perform a special activity. Every organ has one or more specific functions. Which kinds of tissue combine to form the heart? Cardiac Muscle tissue

areolar
epithelium

5. A system is a group of organs working together to perform a special function. Fill in the chart on the next page, listing the organs and function for each body system.

6. The body is divided into cavities containing organs. In which cavity is each of the following organs found?

A. Spinal cord
Spinal Cavity

B. Brain
cranial Cavity

C. Lungs
thoracic Cavity

D. Bladder
pelvic cavity

E. Stomach
abdominal cavity

F. Gallbladder
abdominal cavity

G. Kidneys abdominal cavity

H. Heart thoracic cavity

I. Appendix pelvic cavity

J. Spleen abdominal cavity

K. Uterus pelvic cavity

L. Intestines abdominal cavity

SYSTEM	ORGANS	FUNCTION
Muscular	Muscles	
Skeletal	Bones	
Circulatory	blood heart blood vessels lymphatics and	Lymph Nodes
Digestive	Mouth esophagus stomach Intestines Pharynx	Accessory Organs → Tongue, salivary, appendix glands, teeth, liver gall bladder, pancreas
Respiratory	Nose Pharynx bronchi larynx trachea Lungs	
Urinary	2 Kidneys 2 ureters, urinary meatus bladder, uretha	
Reproductive	Tubes Female Ovaries, vagina, breasts Uterus, Vulva Male Testes, epididymides, semina ducts Penis, ejaculatory ducts, uretha	
Endocrine	Pituitary Parathyroid glands Thymus Pineal gland ? Adrenal glands Islands of Langerhans Placenta	
Nervous	autonomic nervous system cranial and spinal Nerves brain and spinal cord	

7. Here are some definitions you should know. Circle the number of the correct answer.

A. The exchange of gases (oxygen and carbon dioxide) from the air sacs in the lungs through the walls of blood vessels is called

(1) Diffusion.
(2) Osmosis.
(3) Contractility.

B. The production of different kinds of substances from materials in the blood is called

(1) Secretion.
(2) Excretion.
(3) Metabolism.

C. The combining of food and oxygen within a cell is called

(1) Phagocytosis.
(2) Digestion.
(3) Oxidation.

D. Chemicals contained in the water content of the body are called

(1) Ameboids.
(2) Electrolytes.
(3) Fluid-electrolyte balance.

E. The ability of a cell to become shorter and thicker in response to a stimulus is called

(1) Contractility.
(2) Conduction.
(3) Permeability.

Chapter 11

THE SKIN

REFERENCES

Anthony, C. P.: Structure and Function of the Body, pp. 15-18.
Culver, V.: Modern Bedside Nursing, Chapters 6 and 16.
Hoffman, C. P., Lipkin, G., and Thompson, E.: Simplified Nursing, pp. 91-92.
Manner, H.: Elements of Anatomy and Physiology, p. 190.
Memmler, R. L.: The Human Body in Health and Disease, Chapter 12.
Rapier, D. K., et al.: Practical Nursing, p. 68.
Rasmussen, S.: Foundations of Practical and Vocational Nursing, pp. 343-345.
Thompson, E., and Murphy, C.: Textbook of Basic Nursing, pp. 126-128.

1. Color the parts of the skin (Figure 2):

   A. Epidermis - pink

   B. Dermis - blue

   C. Subcutaneous tissue - yellow

2. Label the parts of the skin:

   A. Sebaceous gland

   B. Sweat gland

   C. Arrector muscle

   D. Hair root

   E. Sebaceous duct

3. List the functions of the skin.

4. What causes pimples?

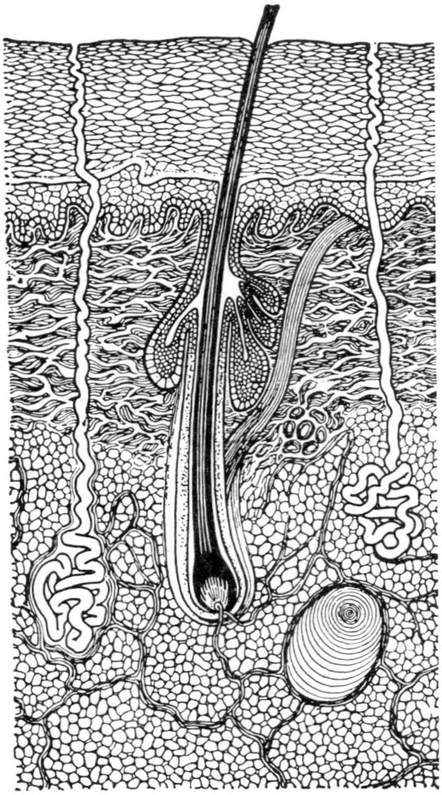

Fig. 2. The Skin. Modified from Tuttle and Schottelius, and Anthony, C. P.: Structure and Function of the Body. 3rd ed. St. Louis, The C. V. Mosby Co., 1968.

5. Discuss the proper hygiene of the skin.

6. What are pores?

7. What are the functions of the nerves in the skin?

8. Discuss the statement, "Two gray hairs come in for every one that is pulled out."

9. Why does one feel uncomfortable in hot humid weather?

10. Describe the structure of the nails and hair.

Chapter 12

THE SKELETAL SYSTEM

REFERENCES

Anthony, C. P.: Structure and Function of the Body, Chapter 2.
Culver, V.: Modern Bedside Nursing, Chapter 7.
Dienhart, C. M.: Basic Human Anatomy and Physiology, Chapter 2.
Hoffman, C. P., Lipkin, G., and Thompson, E.: Simplified Nursing, Chapter 10.
Manner, H.: Elements of Anatomy and Physiology, Chapter 4.
Memmler, R. L.: The Human Body in Health and Disease, Chapter 6.
Rapier, D. K., et al.: Practical Nursing, Chapter 10.
Rasmussen, S.: Foundations of Practical and Vocational Nursing, Chapter 30.
Thompson, E., and Murphy, C.: Textbook of Basic Nursing, Chapter 13.

1. Describe the composition of bones.

2. List the functions of the skeletal system.

3. Label several of the various types of bones in Figure 3 with color. Color:

   A. Long bones - red

   B. Short bones - green

   C. Flat bones - yellow

   D. Irregular bones - blue

4. On the same diagram

   A. Draw:

   (1) A dark red circle around a hinge joint.
   (2) A dark blue circle around a ball-and-socket joint.

   B. Label:

(1) Clavicle	(7) Femur	(13) Tarsals
(2) Scapula	(8) Patella	(14) Carpus
(3) Humerus	(9) Tibia	(15) Metatarsals
(4) Radius	(10) Fibula	(16) Phalanges
(5) Ulna	(11) Vertebrae	(17) Metacarpals
(6) Sternum	(12) Pelvis	(18) Ribs

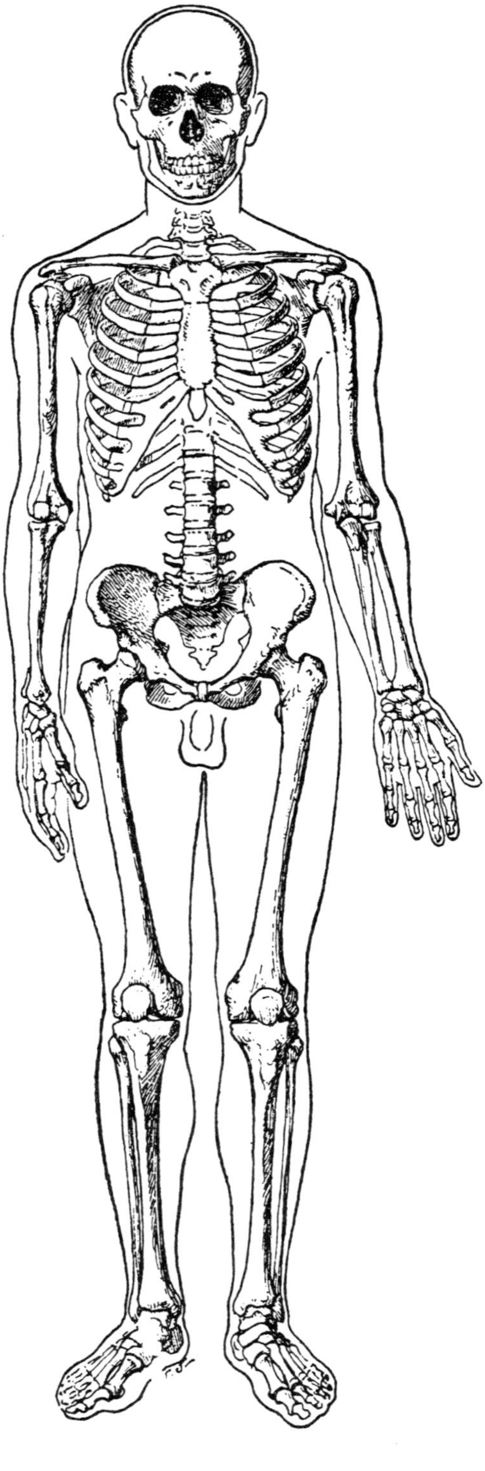

Fig. 3. The skeleton, front view. (Jones and Shepard: Manual of Surgical Anatomy.)

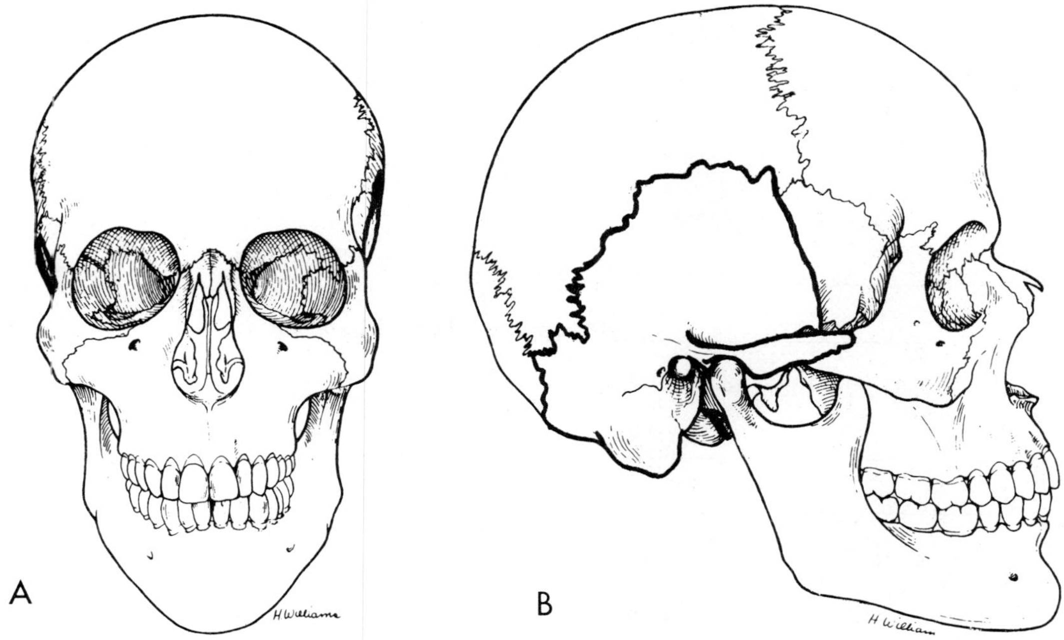

Fig. 4. A. Front view of skull. B. Lateral view of skull. (Francis, C., Knowlton, G., and Tuttle, W.: Textbook of Anatomy and Physiology for Nurses. St. Louis, The C.V. Mosby Co., 1943.)

5. Label the bones of the skull with color. Color:

   A. Frontal - blue
   B. Parietal, lacrimal, zygomatic - gray
   C. Temporal, nasal, mandibular - pink
   D. Maxillary - green
   E. Sphenoidal, occipital - white

6. Complete.

A. The ______________ on the ends of bones forms a padded covering for easy movement.

B. Strong, fibrous bands called ______________ hold bones together. Strong, fibrous bands that hold muscles together are called ______________.

C. The ______________ is the only movable facial bone.

D. The ______________ supports the head and protects the ______ cord. This column is divided into five sections: the ______________, ______________, ______________, ______________ and ______________.

E. The longest and strongest bone in the body is the ______________.

F. When turning one's palm forward and backward, the ______________ crosses the ______________.

G. Cavities in the cranial bones are called ______________.

H. At birth, bones are partly cartilage and do not become hard until approximately ______________ years of age.

I. Proper care of the skeletal system includes: ______________ ______________, ______________ and ______________ ______________.

J. The four curves formed by the vertebrae are the ______________, ______________, ______________, and ______________.

7. Match the movement of the part with the correct term.

	Term	Movement
_____	a. Flexion	1. Away from the midline of the body
_____	b. Extension	2. Towards midline of body
_____	c. Supination	3. Bending the knee
_____	d. Pronation	4. Twisting—as in twisting the head
_____	e. Rotation	5. Straightening the knee
_____	f. Abduction	6. Palms down
_____	g. Adduction	7. Palms up

Chapter 13

THE MUSCULAR SYSTEM

REFERENCES

Anthony, C. P.: Structure and Function of the Body, Chapter 3.
Culver, V.: Modern Bedside Nursing, Chapter 8.
Dienhart, C. M.: Basic Human Anatomy and Physiology, Chapter 3.
Hoffman, C. P., Lipkin, G., and Thompson, E.: Simplified Nursing, Chapter 10.
Manner, H.: Elements of Anatomy and Physiology, Chapter 5.
Memmler, R. L.: The Human Body in Health and Disease, Chapter 6.
Rapier, D. K., et al.: Practical Nursing, Chapter 10.
Rasmussen, S.: Foundations of Practical and Vocational Nursing, Chapter 31.
Thompson, E., and Murphy, C.: Textbook of Basic Nursing, Chapter 13.

---

1. List the functions of the muscular system.

2. How do muscles obtain energy to function?

3. What are the two types of muscle control? Give an example of each.

4. Practice the following exercises used for improving muscle tone and list the groups of muscles which are affected:

   A. Stand on tiptoes several times.

   B. Standing, place both arms at sides. Raise both arms to shoulder height and then lower. Repeat this several times.

5. Define body mechanics.

6. Explain how good body mechanics can be used when doing the following:

   A. Picking up an object from the floor

   B. Writing while sitting at a desk

   C. Standing

   D. Walking

   E. Removing a heavy object from a low shelf

7. Label the following muscles shown in Figure 5.

   A. Deltoideus
   B. Biceps brachii
   C. Triceps brachii
   D. Intercostales
   E. Gluteus maximum
   F. Tibialis anterior
   G. Quadriceps femoris
   H. Gastrocnemius
   I. Sternocleidomastoideus
   J. Latissimus dorsi

8. Draw small red circles where the three common sites of hernia are located. Write in the names of these areas in red.

9. Complete.

   A. Muscles which guard openings of the body by opening and closing are called ________________.

   B. The ____________, a large dome-shaped muscle, aids the ______________ ________ muscles in movements of respiration.

   C. Muscles used as sites for intramuscular injections are the ______________ ________ and ______________.

   D. Specialists who work with injured or inactive muscles in order to reestablish muscular activity are called ____________________.

E. A back rub is comforting to a patient because ________________ on the ________________ in the muscles makes them ________________.

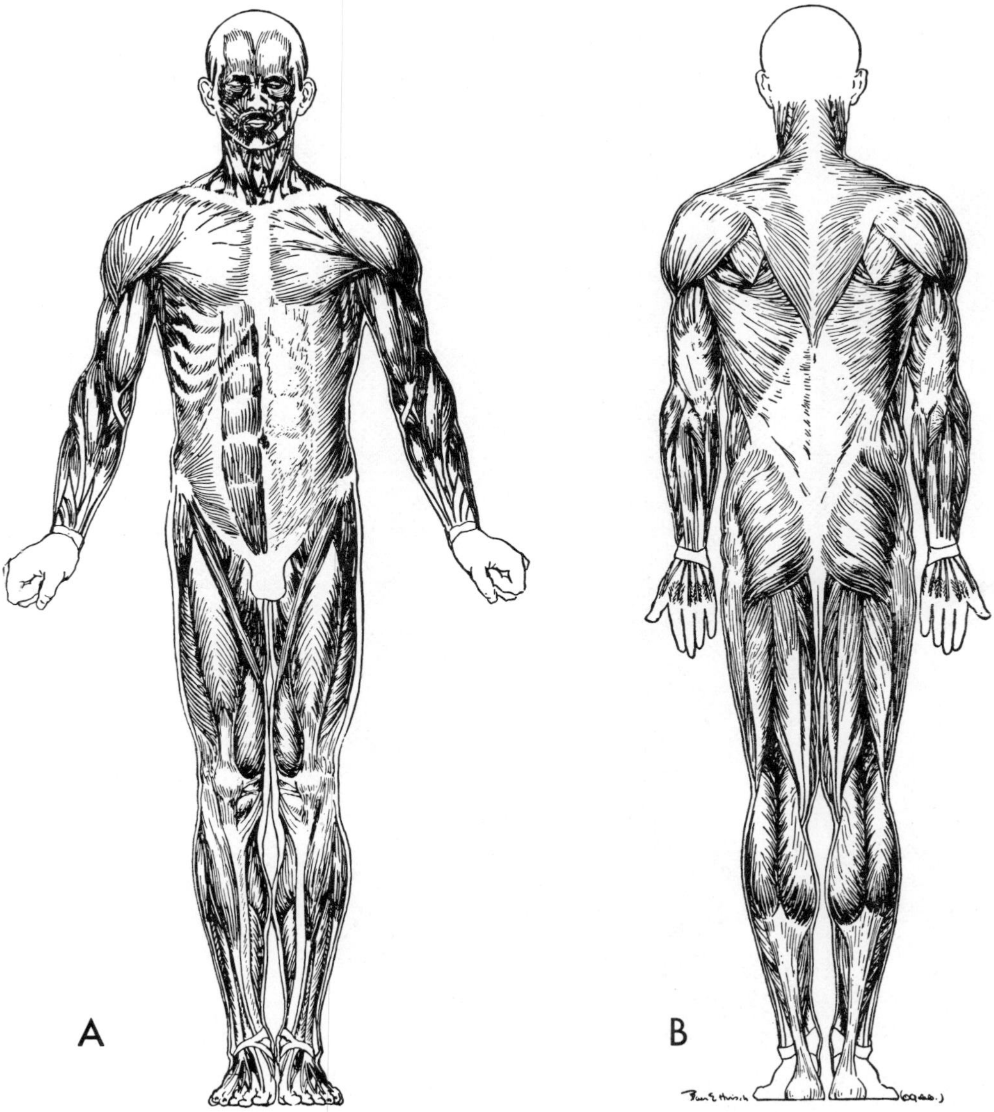

Fig. 5A. Muscles of the body, front view. Fig. 5B. Muscles of the body, back view.

(Thompson, E., and LeBaron, M.: Simplified Nursing. 7th ed. Philadelphia, J.B. Lippincott Co., 1960.)

Chapter 14

THE CIRCULATORY SYSTEM

REFERENCES

Anthony, C. P.: Structure and Function of the Body, Chapter 5.
Culver, V.: Modern Bedside Nursing, Chapter 10.
Dienhart, C. M.: Basic Human Anatomy and Physiology, Chapter 5.
Hoffman, C., Lipkin, G., and Thompson, E.: Simplified Nursing, Chapter 11.
Manner, H.: Elements of Anatomy and Physiology, Chapter 7.
Memmler, R. L.: The Human Body in Health and Disease, Chapters 6-9.
Rapier, D. K., et al.: Practical Nursing, pp. 55-58.
Rasmussen, S.: Foundations of Practical and Vocational Nursing, Chapter 33.
Thompson, E., and Murphy, C.: Textbook of Basic Nursing, Chapter 15.

---

1. List the functions of each part of the circulatory system.

PART	FUNCTIONS
Heart	
Blood	
Arteries	
Veins	
Capillaries	
Lymphatics	

2. Complete.

The blood is composed of liquids and solids. The liquid substance is called ____________________, and its function is to carry ______________________________. The solids are red blood cells, white blood cells and platelets. The red blood cells contain _________________, a substance which gives the cells a red color and which carries ____________________ to the body cells. The average number of red cells in the blood is _______________ per cubic millimeter. The white blood cells, which average in number from ____________ to ____________ per cubic millimeter, protect the body against ____________ . When an infection is present in the body, the number of white blood cells ________________. One of the functions of the platelets is to help in ______________ of the blood. The pressure the blood exerts on the walls of the arteries is called ________________. This pressure is measured with a ________________ and is very important in detecting many types of diseases. One inherited blood characteristic is called the ________ factor. Most individuals are Rh ____________ .

3. Label the parts of the heart in Figure 6.

A. Right and left atrium
B. Right and left ventricle
C. Mitral valve
D. Tricuspid valve
E. Pulmonary valve
F. Aortic valve
G. Inferior vena cava
H. Superior vena cava
I. Aorta
J. Pulmonary veins
K. Pulmonary arteries

4. Color:

A. Pericardium - green
B. Endocardium - red
C. Myocardium - blue

5. Describe the difference in structure of

A. Veins
B. Arteries
C. Capillaries

6. The pulse is the rhythmic beating of the heart. The pulse can best be felt in which arteries?

7. What is the normal adult pulse rate?

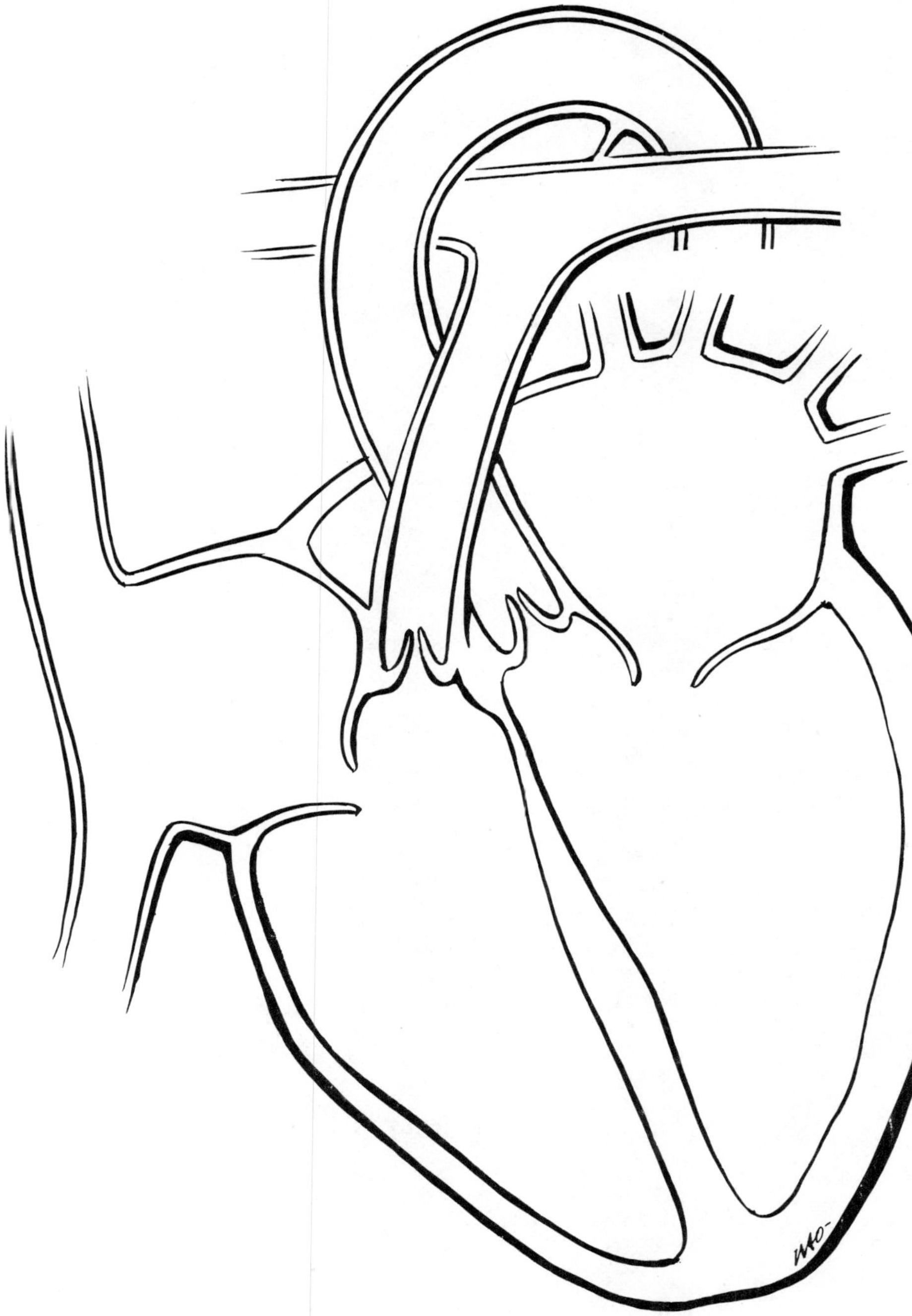

Fig. 6. Heart chambers.

Chapter 15

THE NERVOUS SYSTEM

REFERENCES

Anthony, C. P.: Structure and Function of the Body, Chapter 4.
Culver, V.: Modern Bedside Nursing, Chapter 15.
Dienhart, C. M.: Basic Human Anatomy and Physiology, Chapter 4.
Hoffman, C., Lipkin, G., and Thompson, E.: Simplified Nursing, Chapter 17.
Manner, H.: Elements of Anatomy and Physiology, Chapter 6.
Memmler, R. L.: The Human Body in Health and Disease, Chapter 14.
Rapier, D. K., et al.: Practical Nursing, p. 48.
Rasmussen, S.: Foundations of Practical and Vocational Nursing, Chapter 36.
Thompson, E., and Murphy, C.: Textbook of Basic Nursing, Chapter 14.

1. The functions of the nervous system are:

2. Label the parts of the central nervous system.

   A. Cerebrum
   B. Cerebellum
   C. Pons
   D. Medulla
   E. Spinal cord

3. Color the lobes of the cerebrum:

   A. Frontal - yellow
   B. Parietal - red
   C. Occipital - blue

4. Match Column I with Column II.

Column I	Column II
a. Meninges	____ 1. Removal of small amount of spinal fluid for diagnostic purposes
b. Neuron	____ 2. Nerve cell
c. Lumbar puncture	____ 3. Covering of nerve fibers
d. Autonomic	____ 4. Covering of brain and spinal cord
e. Myelin sheath	____ 5. Part of the nervous system which controls involuntary activity of the body

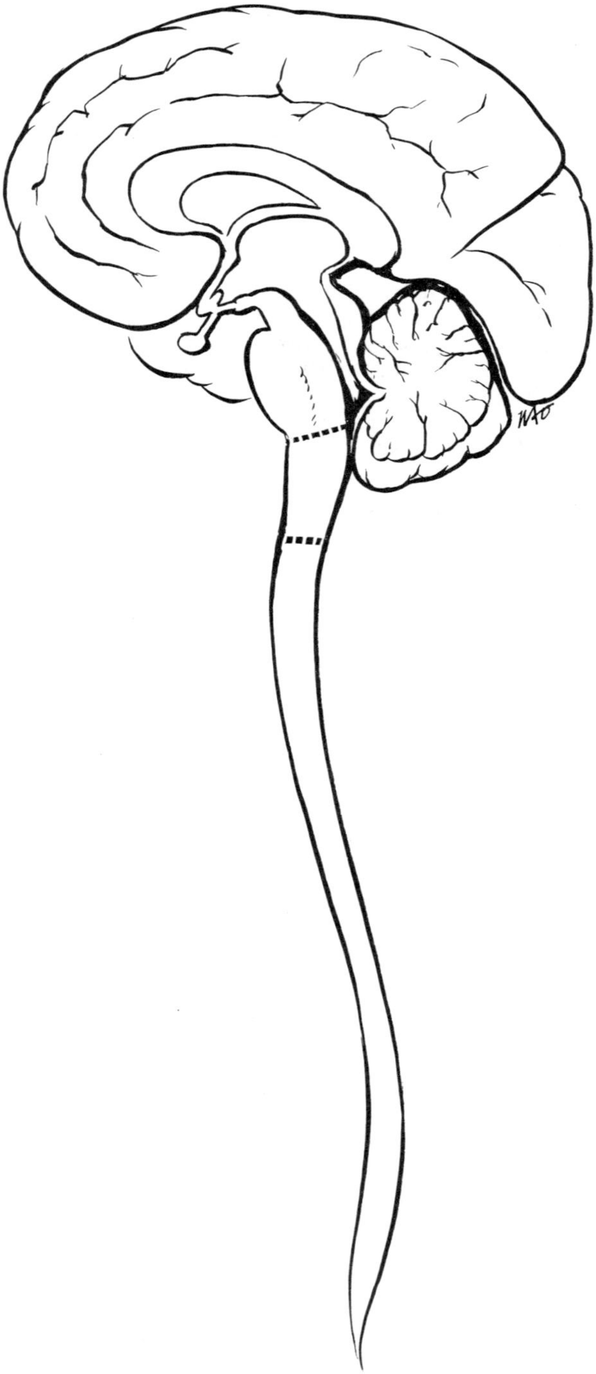

Fig. 7. The central nervous system.

5. Multiple Choice. Circle the correct answer to each question.

A. One function of the spinal cord is to

(1) Control balance and coordination.
(2) Conduct impulses from various nerves to the brain.
(3) Control thinking.

B. The function of the cerebrum is to

(1) Control motor reflexes and senses and record knowledge.
(2) Control balance and coordination.
(3) Connect the cerebral cortex to the medulla.

C. The function of the cerebellum is to

(1) Control balance and coordination.
(2) Record knowledge.
(3) Conduct impulses to the brain.

D. The medulla

(1) Records knowledge.
(2) Influences balance and thinking.
(3) Influences vital activities such as breathing and heartbeat.

E. The pons

(1) Connects the brain to the spinal cord.
(2) Is the most vital reflex center.
(3) Carries messages between the cerebrum and cerebellum.

Chapter 16

THE DIGESTIVE SYSTEM

REFERENCES

Anthony, C. P.: Structure and Function of the Body, Chapter 6.
Culver, V.: Modern Bedside Nursing, Chapter 11.
Dienhart, C. M.: Basic Human Anatomy and Physiology, Chapter 7.
Hoffman, C., Lipkin, G., and Thompson, E.: Simplified Nursing, Chapter 13.
Manner, H.: Elements of Anatomy and Physiology, Chapter 10.
Memmler, R. L.: The Human Body in Health and Disease, Chapter 10.
Rapier, D. K., et al.: Practical Nursing, p. 64.
Rasmussen, S.: Foundations of Practical and Vocational Nursing, Chapter 34.
Thompson, E., and Murphy, C.: Textbook of Basic Nursing, Chapter 17.

1. List the two main functions of the digestive system.

2. List the functions of each part of the digestive system.

PART	FUNCTIONS
Mouth	
Esophagus	
Stomach	
Small Intestine	
Large Intestine	
Gallbladder	
Pancreas	
Liver	

3. Label the parts of a tooth shown in Figure 8 in color. Color:

A. Enamel - white B. Dentine - gray C. Cement - yellow

D. Gum - red E. Canal - green

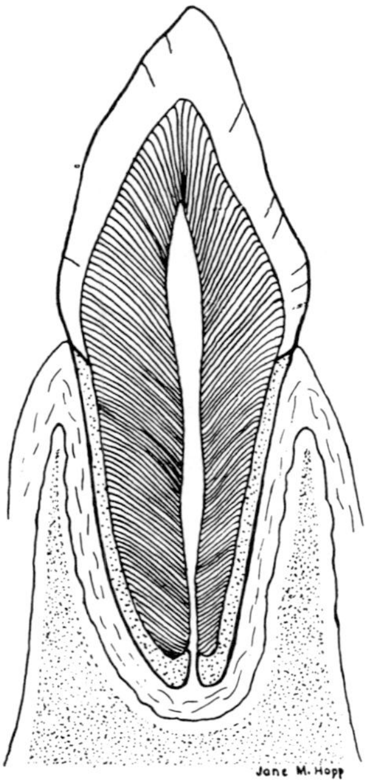

Fig. 8. Vertical section of an incisor tooth. (From Francis, C., Knowlton, G., and Tuttle, W.: Textbook of Anatomy and Physiology for Nurses. St. Louis, The C.V. Mosby Co., 1943.)

4. Label the permanent teeth in Figure 9 in color. Color:

A. Incisors - yellow
B. Canine - white
C. Premolars - red
D. Molars - blue

5. True or False. Circle T if the statement is true; if the statement is false. Correct the statements that are false by crossing out the word or words that are wrong and placing the correct word or words in the space above.

T F 1. The gastrointestinal tract is lined with mucous membrane.

T F 2. The alternation of contracting and relaxing motions in the digestive tube which pushes food along is called mastication.

T F 3. Saliva changes starches to sugar.

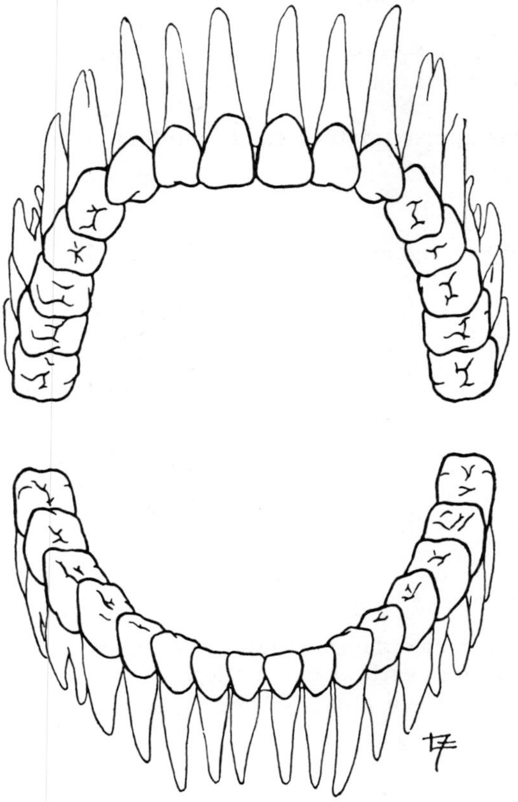

Fig. 9. Permanent Teeth.
(From Miller & Miller: Good Health.)

T F 4. Gastric juice contains insulin and hydrochloric acid.

T F 5. As food passes through the stomach, it enters the part of the small intestine called the ileum.

T F 6. The anus is guarded by internal and external sphincter muscles.

T F 7. Emotions can affect the process of digestion.

T F 8. The process of body cells using food materials is called absorption.

T F 9. The fundus is the lower portion of the stomach which connects to the small intestine.

T F 10. Regular bowel elimination is necessary to maintaining good health.

T F 11. The proper way to brush teeth is to brush down on the lower teeth and up on the upper teeth.

T F 12. The pharynx has a dual function; it is a passageway for air and for food.

T F 13. Bile is necessary for the digestion of starches.

T F 14. If bile cannot pass directly into the small intestine, it is absorbed by the blood and causes a condition known as jaundice.

T F 15. It takes approximately eight hours for food to pass completely through the digestive tract.

6. Label the parts of the digestive system in Figure 10.

A. Esophagus
B. Stomach
C. Liver
D. Pylorus
E. Pancreas
F. Gallbladder
G. Duodenum
H. Ileum
I. Jejunum
J. Appendix
K. Cecum
L. Ascending colon
M. Descending colon
N. Transverse colon
O. Sigmoid colon
P. Rectum

7. Color:

A. Hepatic and pancreatic duct - green
B. Salivary glands and cystic duct - yellow
C. Common bile duct - red

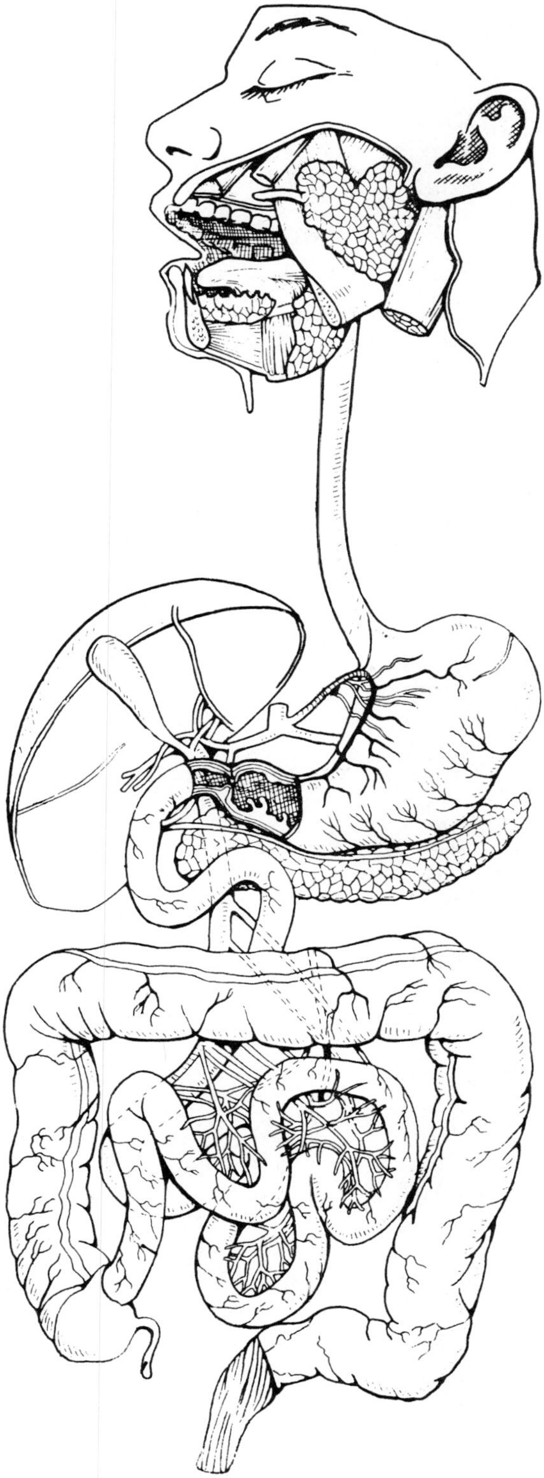

Fig. 10. Digestive system. (Denoyer Geppert Company, Chicago, Illinois.)

Chapter 17

THE RESPIRATORY SYSTEM

REFERENCES

Anthony, C. P.: Structure and Function of the Body, Chapter 7.
Culver, V.: Modern Bedside Nursing, Chapter 9.
Dienhart, C. M.: Basic Human Anatomy and Physiology, Chapter 6.
Hoffman, C., Lipkin, G., and Thompson, E.: Simplified Nursing, Chapter 12.
Manner, H.: Elements of Anatomy and Physiology, Chapter 9.
Memmler, R. L.: The Human Body in Health and Disease, Chapter 11.
Rapier, D. K., et al.: Practical Nursing, p. 59.
Rasmussen, S.: Foundations of Practical and Vocational Nursing, Chapter 32.
Thompson, E., and Murphy, C.: Textbook of Basic Nursing, Chapter 16.

1. List the functions of the respiratory system.

2. List the functions of each part of the respiratory system.

PART	FUNCTION
Nose	
Pharynx	
Larynx	
Trachea	
Bronchi	
Lungs	

3. On the diagram of the respiratory system (Figure 11)

   A. Label:

      (1) Larynx
      (2) Trachea
      (3) Bronchi

(4) Bronchiole
(5) Alveoli

B. Place a green X on the apex of each lung, a red X on the base of each lung and a blue X on the mediastinum.

C. Draw the pleurae with red, the diaphragm with green and the rib cage with brown.

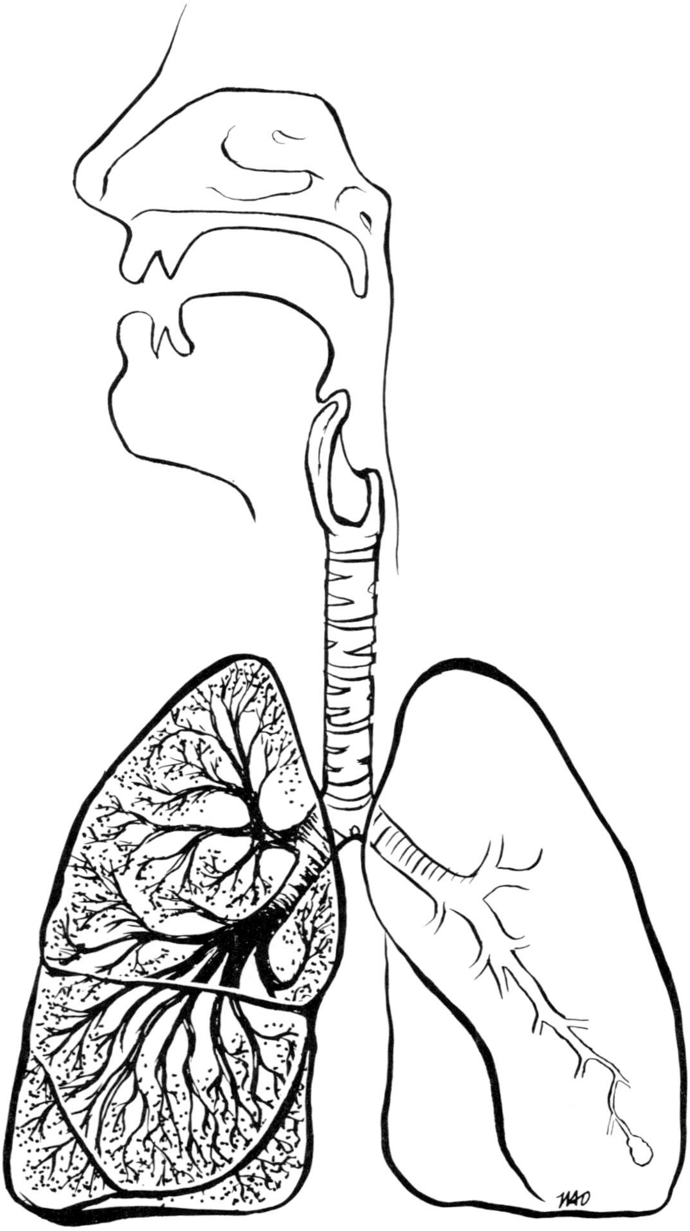

Fig. 11. Respiratory system.

4. Match Column I with Column II.

Column I

a. Epiglottis
b. Expiration
c. Oxygen
d. Sinuses
e. Smell
f. Blood
g. Vocal cords
h. Respiration
i. Carbon dioxide
j. Inhalation

Column II

e 1. Sense perception in nasal passage
c 2. 20 per cent normally found in air
i 3. Excessive amount in body stimulates respiratory center in brain
b 4. Eliminating carbon dioxide
a 5. Prevents choking when eating
d 6. Open into upper part of nasal cavities
j 7. Rib cage expands
g 8. Vibrate to produce sound
h 9. Inhalation and expiration
f 10. Carries oxygen from lungs to parts of body

5. Trace the passage of oxygen through the body from the time it is inhaled to the time it is exhaled. This includes its passage through two body systems, respiratory and circulatory.

Chapter 18

THE URINARY SYSTEM

REFERENCES

Anthony, C. P.: Structure and Function of the Body, Chapter 8.
Culver, V.: Modern Bedside Nursing, Chapter 13.
Dienhart, C. M.: Basic Human Anatomy and Physiology, Chapter 8.
Hoffman, C., Lipkin, G., and Thompson, E.: Simplified Nursing, Chapter 14.
Manner, H.: Elements of Anatomy and Physiology, Chapter 11.
Memmler, R. L.: The Human Body in Health and Disease, Chapter 13.
Rapier, D. K., et al.: Practical Nursing, p. 67.
Rasmussen, S.: Foundations of Practical and Vocational Nursing, Chapter 35.
Thompson, E., and Murphy, C.: Textbook of Basic Nursing, Chapter 18.

1. Label the parts of the urinary system shown in Figure 12 and, under each name, print the function of the part. Label:

   A. Kidney
   B. Ureter
   C. Bladder
   D. Urethra

2. Color:

   A. Renal fundus - blue
   B. Renal pelvis - red

3. Describe the normal characteristics of urine. Why is it important to know these characteristics?

4. What factors influence the amount of urinary output?

5. In what ways can the measurement of fluid intake and output be an aid to the physician?

6. What is the normal daily output of urine?

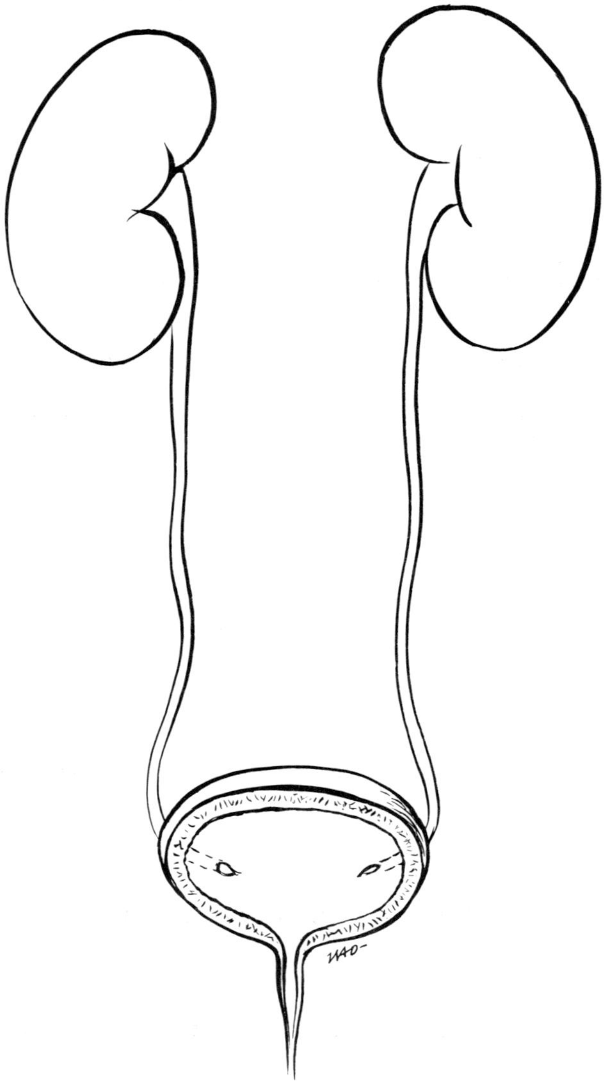

Fig. 12. Urinary system.

7. Complete.

The urinary system, along with the ______________________ , ____________________ and ____________________________ systems, eliminates waste from the body. The substance which the urinary system excretes is called ________________. This process is accomplished by a group of several organs. The kidneys are composed of many tiny ________________ which filter the blood. The______________, about ten inches long, extend from the _______________ of the kidney to the ______________________. The bladder is a sac lined with ______________________ and holds about __________________ of urine. Elimination of urine from the bladder is voluntarily controlled by the _____________________.

8. Match Column I with Column II.

Column I	Column II
___ a. Renal fascia	1. Fibrous covering of kidney
___ b. Cortex	2. Coiled tube connected to capillary cluster in neuron
___ c. Medulla	3. Inner portion of kidney
___ d. Glomerulus	4. Outer portion of kidney
___ e. Convoluted tubule	5. Capillary cluster in nephron

Chapter 19

THE REPRODUCTIVE SYSTEM

REFERENCES

Anthony, C. P.: Structure and Function of the Body, Chapter 9.
Culver, V.: Modern Bedside Nursing, Chapter 13.
Dienhart, C. M.: Basic Human Anatomy and Physiology, Chapter 10.
Hoffman, C., Lipkin, G., and Thompson, E.: Simplified Nursing, Chapter 15.
Manner, H.: Elements of Anatomy and Physiology, Chapter 11.
Memmler, R. L.: The Human Body in Health and Disease, Chapter 17.
Rapier, D. K., et al.: Practical Nursing, Chapter 13.
Rasmussen, S.: Foundations of Practical and Vocational Nursing, Chapter 39.
Thompson, E., and Murphy, C.: Textbook of Basic Nursing, Chapter 19.

THE FEMALE REPRODUCTIVE SYSTEM

1. Color the parts of the adult female reproductive system shown in Figure 13.

   A. Color:

      (1) Uterus - pink
      (2) Ovaries - blue
      (3) Vagina - green
      (4) Fallopian tubes - yellow

   B. Label:

      (1) Cervix
      (2) Fundus
      (3) Cervical canal

2. Color the block preceding each statement to match the part in Figure 13 which the statement describes.

   ☐ A. Contains thousands of egg cells at birth. These cells do not mature until puberty.
   ☐ B. A hollow, muscular, pear-shaped organ located in the center of the pelvic cavity.
   ☐ C. Receptacle for sperm cells during intercourse.
   ☐ D. Place where sperm cell meets ovum.
   ☐ E. Lined with mucous membrane called endometrium.
   ☐ F. Secretes the hormones estrone and progesterone.
   ☐ G. Opens into the peritoneal cavity.
   ☐ H. The lower part of the birth canal.
   ☐ I. The fertilized ovum attaches to its walls and grows, establishing pregnancy.
   ☐ J. Contains graafian follicles

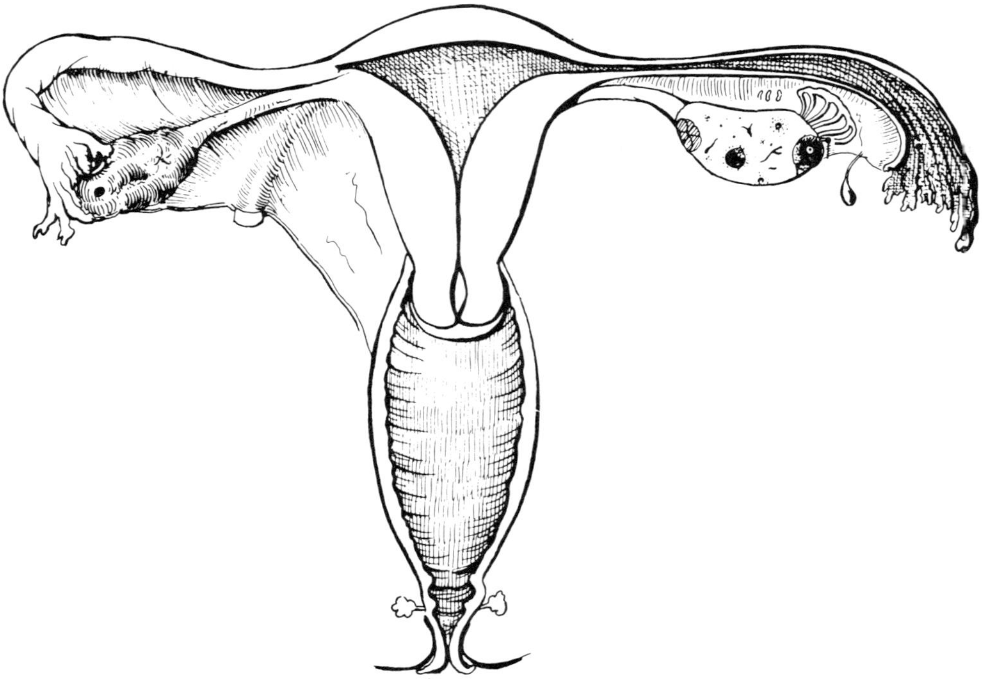

Fig. 13. Female reproductive organs. (Denoyer-Geppert Company, Chicago, Illinois.)

3. Label the parts of the female genitalia in Figure 14.

   A. Labia majora
   B. Labia minora
   C. Clitoris
   D. Urinary meatus
   E. Vagina

4. Explain the anatomical structure of the breasts.

5. What change takes place in the areola during pregnancy?

6. Explain the action of the following hormones during the menstrual cycle.

   A. Pituitary hormone
   B. Estrogen
   C. Progesterone

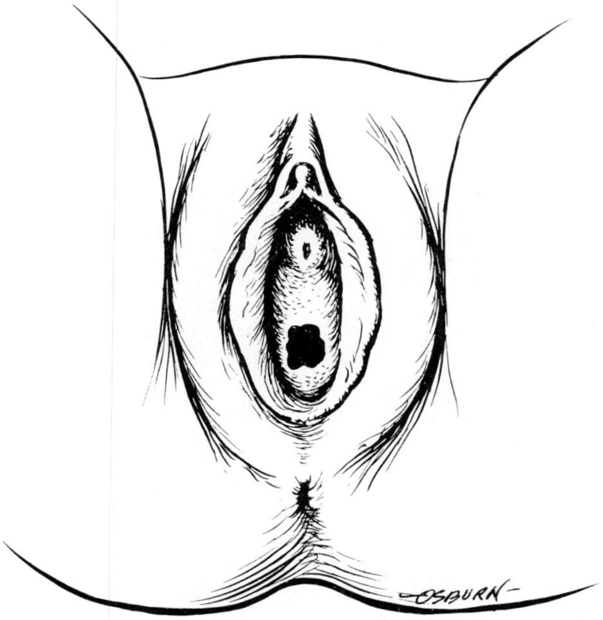

Fig. 14. External female genitalia.

7. Match the changes which take place in the female reproductive system during the menstrual cycle with the time that each usually takes place.

Time	Changes
_____ a. 7-10 days after menstrual flow ceases	1. Ovulation occurs
_____ b. 14 days after beginning of menstrual flow	2. Graafian follicle and ovum are maturing
_____ c. 18-20 days after beginning of menstrual flow	3. If no fertilization occurs, endometrium diminishes followed by sloughing.
	4. Endometrium thickens
	5. Pregnancy can occur

THE MALE REPRODUCTIVE SYSTEM

1. Label the parts of the male reproductive system shown in Figure 15.

   A. Scrotum
   B. Testes
   C. Epididymis
   D. Seminal duct
   E. Seminal vesicle
   F. Prostate gland
   G. Urethra
   H. Penis

2. Describe the dual function of the male urethra.

3. Define:

   A. Phimosis

   B. Copulation

   C. Circumcision

   D. Gonads

   E. Gamete

   F. Zygote

   G. Spermatozoa

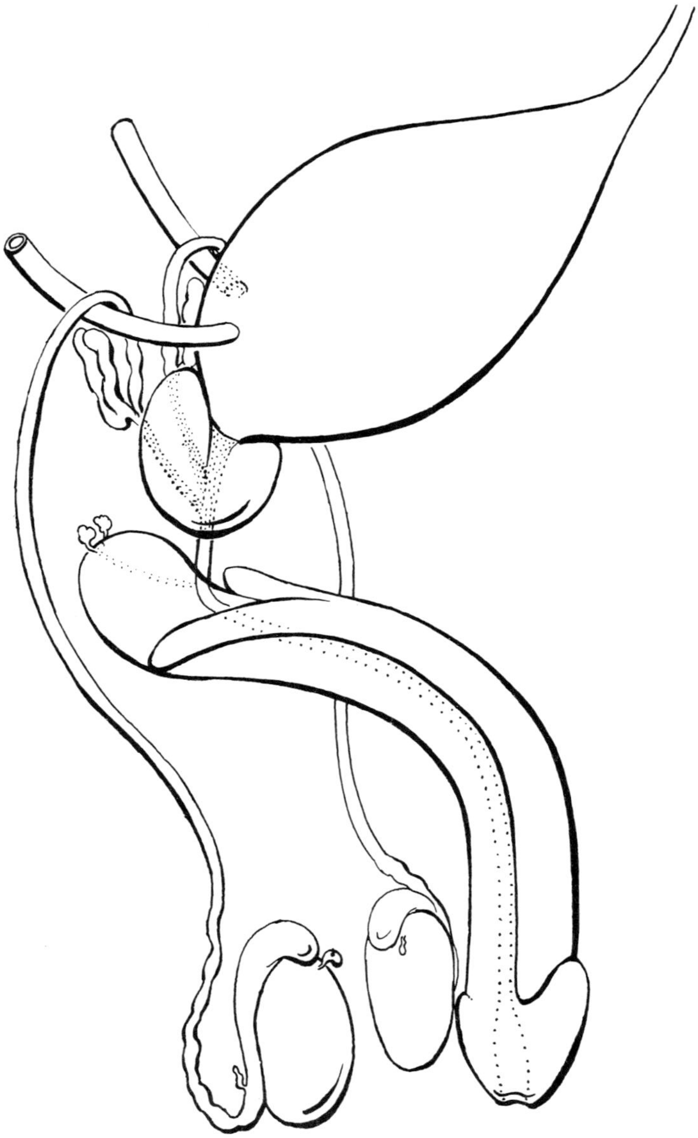

Fig. 15. Male reproductive organs. (Denoyer-Geppert Company, Chicago, Illinois.)

Chapter 20

THE ENDOCRINE SYSTEM

REFERENCES

Anthony, C. P.: Structure and Function of the Body, Chapter 10.
Culver, V.: Modern Bedside Nursing, Chapter 14.
Dienhart, C. M.: Basic Human Anatomy and Physiology, Chapter 9.
Hoffman, C., Lipkin, G., and Thompson, E.: Simplified Nursing, Chapter 16.
Manner, H.: Elements of Anatomy and Physiology, Chapter 8.
Rapier, D. K., et al.: Practical Nursing, Chapter 12.
Rasmussen, S.: Foundations of Practical and Vocational Nursing, Chapter 38.
Thompson, E., and Murphy, C.: Textbook of Basic Nursing, Chapter 20.

1. Briefly describe the endocrine system.

2. What substances do the endocrine glands secrete?

3. What are the functions of the endocrine system?

4. Label the parts of the endocrine system shown in Figure 16.

   A. Thyroid
   B. Parathyroid
   C. Pineal
   D. Pituitary
   E. Thymus
   F. Adrenal
   G. Pancreas
   H. Gonads

5. Which endocrine gland helps to control many of the other endocrine glands?

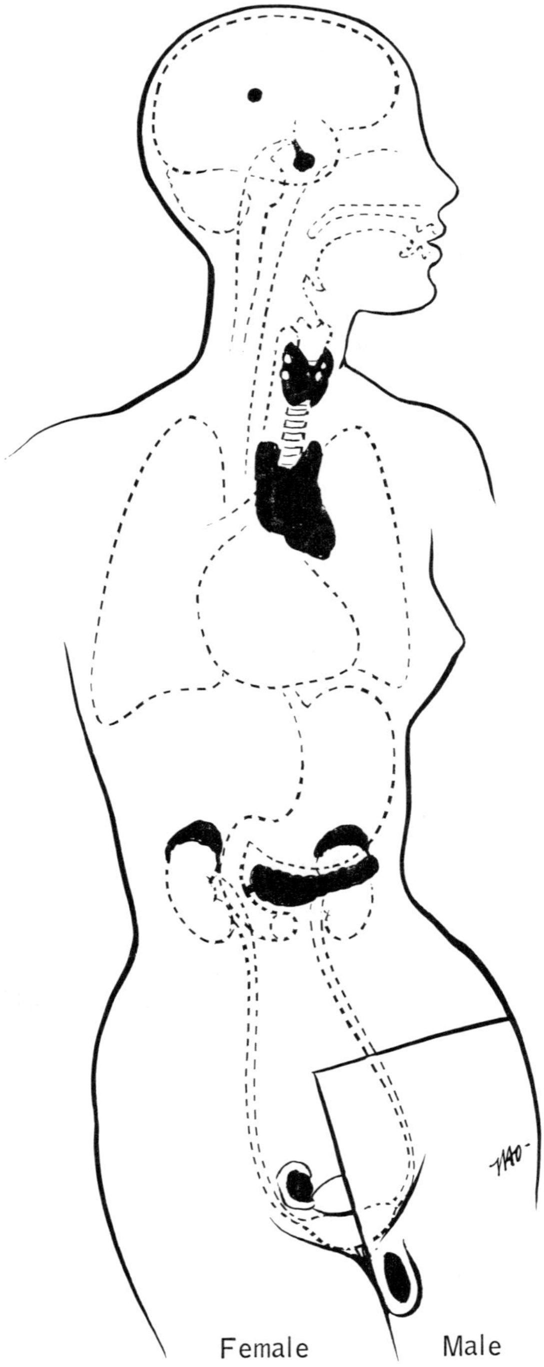

Fig. 16. Endocrine glands.

6. Define:

   A. Hypofunction

   B. Hyperfunction

7. Name a temporary endocrine gland. What is its possible function?

8. Describe the size of the parathyroid glands.

9. What disease results from too little insulin in the body?

10. Complete the table.

GLAND	FUNCTION	HORMONE (S) SECRETED
Pituitary		
Thyroid		
Parathyroid		
Adrenal		
Pancreas		
Gonads		

Chapter 21

THE SPECIAL SENSES

REFERENCES

Anthony, C. P.: Structure and Function of the Body, pp. 59-62.
Culver, V.: Modern Bedside Nursing, Chapter 16.
Dienhart, C. M.: Basic Human Anatomy and Physiology, pp. 87-91.
Hoffman, C., Lipkin, G., and Thompson, E.: Simplified Nursing, pp. 135-137.
Manner, H.: Elements of Anatomy and Physiology, Chapter 6.
Memmler, R. L.: The Human Body in Health and Disease, Chapter 15.
Rapier, D. K., et al.: Practical Nursing, pp. 52-54.
Rasmussen, S.: Foundations of Practical and Vocational Nursing, Chapter 37.
Thompson, E., and Murphy, C.: Textbook of Basic Nursing, Chapter 31.

THE EAR

1. Label the parts of the ear in Figure 17.

   A. Color:

   (1) External ear - blue
   (2) Internal ear - pink

   B. Label:

   (1) Pinna
   (2) Auditory canal
   (3) Tympanic membrane
   (4) Malleus
   (5) Anvil
   (6) Stirrup
   (7) Cochlea
   (8) Eustachian tube

2. Describe how sound waves travel through the ear from the time they are picked up by the pinna to the time they reach the hearing center in the brain.

3. What is the dual function of the internal ear?

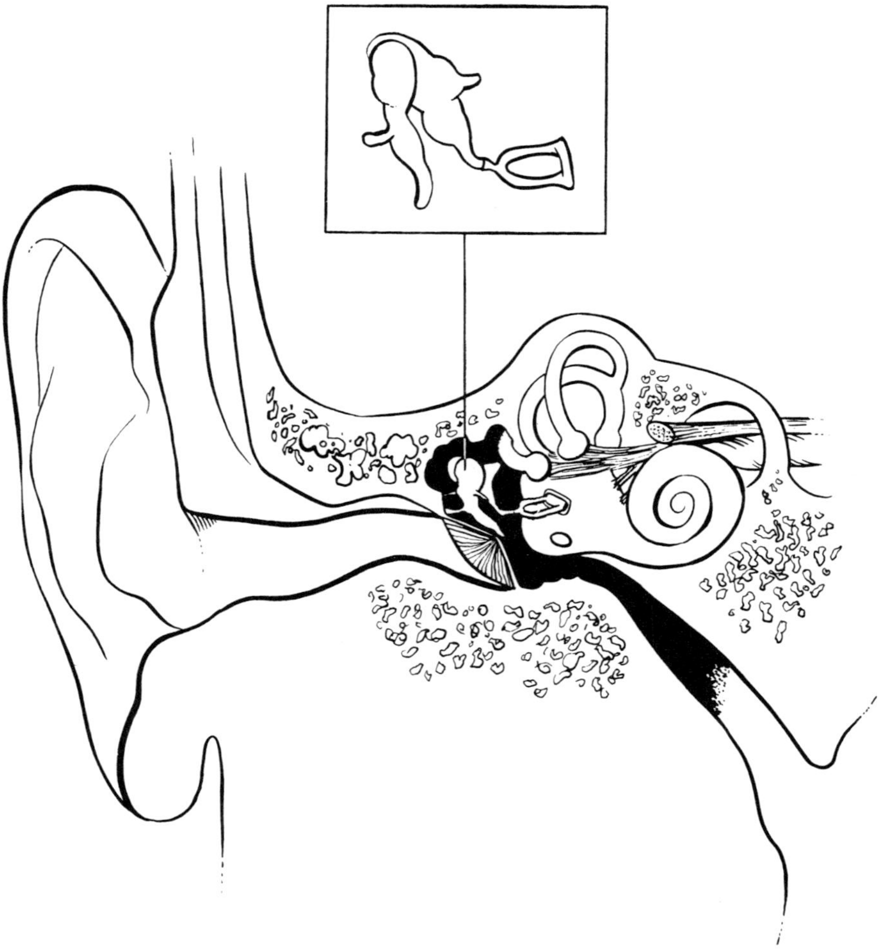

Fig. 17. The human ear. (McKean, I.: Anatomy and Physiology Laboratory Manual and Study Guide.)

4. What anatomic structure makes it easy for a throat infection to spread to the middle ear?

THE EYE

1. Label the parts of the eye in Figure 18.

A. Color:

(1) Retina - red
(2) Sclera - blue
(3) Choroid - yellow
(4) Extrinsic muscles - brown

B. Label:

(1) Iris
(2) Cornea
(3) Ciliary muscle
(4) Optic nerve
(5) Blind spot
(6) Lens

(7) Pupil
(8) Aqueous humor
(9) Vitreous humor

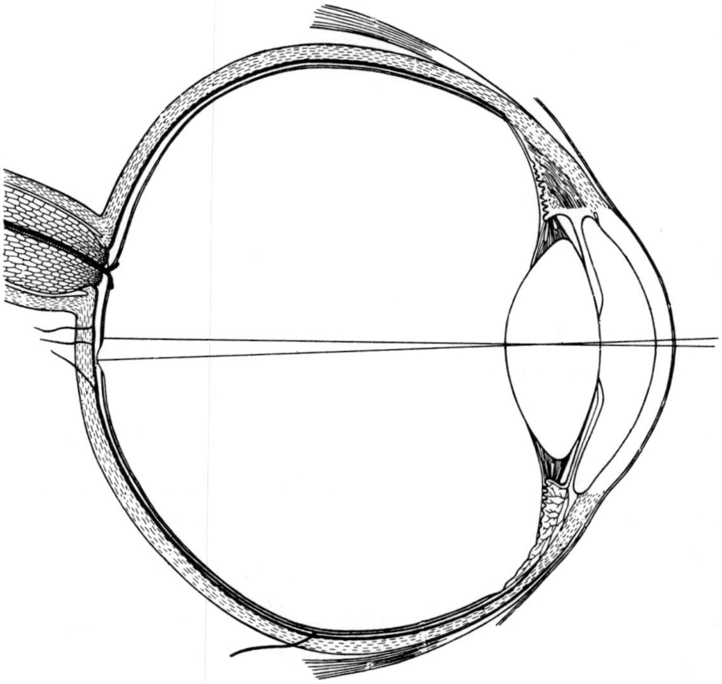

Fig. 18. The human eye. (Courtesy, General Biological Supply House, Inc., Chicago, Illinois.)

2. Describe how light rays travel through the eye from the time they enter the cornea to the time they reach the sight center in the brain.

3. Give the function of each of the following parts:

   A. Conjunctiva

   B. Lacrimal apparatus

   C. Eyelids

   D. Eye muscles

4. Match Column I with Column II.

Column I	Column II
a. Optician	____ 1. Ability of eye to focus light rays according to distance of object
b. Ophthalmologist	____ 2. Myopia
c. Farsightedness	____ 3. Artificial lenses
d. Nearsightedness	____ 4. Cloudy lenses
e. Eyeglasses	____ 5. A specialist in eye diseases
f. Binocular	____ 6. A person licensed to fit eyeglasses according to a prescription
g. Cataract	____ 7. Pertaining to two eyes
h. Astigmatism	____ 8. Light focuses on more than one point in retina
i. Accommodation	____ 9. Light rays focus behind retina

5. Fill in the blanks:

   The ____________ cells are the sensory receptors for the sense of smell. The sense of smell is closely related to the sense of taste. The receptors for taste are called ____________ ____________ . Additional general senses include ____________ , ____________ and ____________ .

PART IV

NUTRITION AND DIET THERAPY

Chapter 22

PRINCIPLES OF GOOD NUTRITION

OUR FOOD NEEDS

CLASSIFICATION OF FOODS

UTILIZATION OF FOODS

REFERENCES

Culver, V.: Modern Bedside Nursing, Chapter 25.
Hoffman, C., Lipkin, G., and Thompson, E.: Simplified Nursing, pp. 141-152.
Howe, P. S.: Nutrition for Practical Nurses. 4th ed. Philadelphia, W. B. Saunders Co., 1967, Chapters 1 to 7.
Mowry, L.: Basic Nutrition and Diet Therapy for Practical Nurses. 3rd ed. St. Louis, The C. V. Mosby Co., 1966, Chapters 1 to 3.
Rapier, D. K., et al.: Practical Nursing, Chapter 36.
Shackelton, A. D.: Practical Nurse Nutrition Education. 2nd ed. Philadelphia, W. B. Saunders Co., 1966, Chapters 1 to 4.
Thompson, E., and Murphy, C.: Textbook of Basic Nursing, Chapter 22.

---

1. Review Chapter 16.

2. Define:

   A. Nutrition

   B. Nutrients

   C. Dietetics

   D. Dietitian

3. List the three functions of food in the body.

4. List five characteristics of a well nourished body.

5. List the daily requirements of each of the four basic food groups.

   A. Milk Group

      (1) Children:_______ cups

      (2) Adolescents:_______ cups

      (3) Adults: _______ cups

      (4) Pregnant women: _______ cups

   B. Meat Group

      (1) Meats, poultry, eggs: ____________ servings

      (2) Alternate foods: ______________________________

   C. Vegetable-Fruit Group

      (1) Total daily servings: ___________________

      (2) Dark yellow and dark green vegetables are needed ____________________ day.

      (3) Citrus fruits:____________ servings per day.

   D. Bread-Cereal Group: ____________ servings per day.

6. Complete the table.

Nutrient	Functions
Carbohydrates	
Fats	
Minerals	
Proteins	
Vitamins	
Water	

Carbohydrate sources include sugars and starches. There are several kinds of sugars.

7. Match Column I with Column II.

Column I		Column II
a. Glucose	B	1. Found in milk
b. Lactose	D	2. Product of sprouting grains
c. Sucrose	A	3. Only form of sugar ready for body use
d. Maltose	E	4. Found mostly in fruits and honey
e. Fructose	C	5. Form of sugar used on table

8. What are the sources of starch?

9. Discuss the importance of cellulose in the diet.

10. What is the nutritional value of cellulose?

11. List some foods high in cellulose content.

12. What is glycogen?

Fats are found in animals and plants.

13. Match Column I with Column II.

Column I		Column II
a. Visible fats	B	1. Product of fat metabolism
b. Fatty acids	A	2. Examples are butter, lard, oils
c. Acetone bodies	E	3. Type of fat consistency
d. Cholesterol	C	4. Linoleic, linolenic, arachidonic
e. Unsaturated	D	5. Combination of fatty acids and alcohols found in all body tissue

14. How is margarine made?

Proteins come from animal and plant food sources.

15. Complete the table.

Proteins	Function	Sources
Complete		
Partially complete		
Incomplete		

16. What percentage of the daily caloric intake should be made up of proteins?

Minerals have a number of food sources. Important aspects in selecting foods containing minerals are to select the food highest in a particular mineral content and to select the mineral in a form the body can readily use and store.

17. Complete the table.

Mineral	Function	Sources
Calcium		
Phosphorus		
Iron		
Iodine		

18. Vitamins are found in a variety of plant and animal food sources. They are eight vitamins necessary for health. What are the best food sources of the following vitamins:

A. Vitamin A (carotene):

B. Vitamin B complex

(1) Thiamine (B_1):

(2) Riboflavin (B_2):

(3) Niacin (nicotinic acid):

C. Vitamin C:

D. Vitamin D:

E. Vitamin K:

F. Vitamin E:

19. Explain the digestion and absorption process of each of the following food nutrients:

A. Carbohydrates

B. Fats

C. Proteins

20. What is meant by a "fortified" or "enriched" food?

21. Which food nutrients are added to commercially prepared foods?

22. What should be the daily intake of water?

23. Name three characteristics of vitamins which are important in selecting methods of storing and cooking them.

24. What factors influence the daily caloric requirements of the body?

25. If you were served a daily diet containing 114 grams carbohydrates, 75 grams protein and 45 grams fat, what would the caloric value be? Would this daily diet contain enough calories to supply the energy you need?

26. Define obesity and discuss its cause in relation to caloric intake.

Chapter 23

SELECTION, CARE AND SERVING OF FOODS

REFERENCES

Hoffman, C., Lipkin, G., and Thompson, E.: Simplified Nursing, pp. 152-158.
Howe, P. S.: Nutrition for Practical Nurses, Chapters 10-13, Section III.
Mowry, L.: Basic Nutrition and Diet Therapy for Nurses, Chapters 11-13.
Rapier, D. K., et al.: Practical Nursing, Chapter 38.
Shackelton, A. D.: Practical Nurse Nutrition Education, Unit 3.
Thompson, E., and Murphy, C.: Textbook of Basic Nursing, Chapter 24.

1. How may nationality or religion influence the diet? Give examples.

2. Write the number of each article in its proper place on the tray shown in Figure 19.

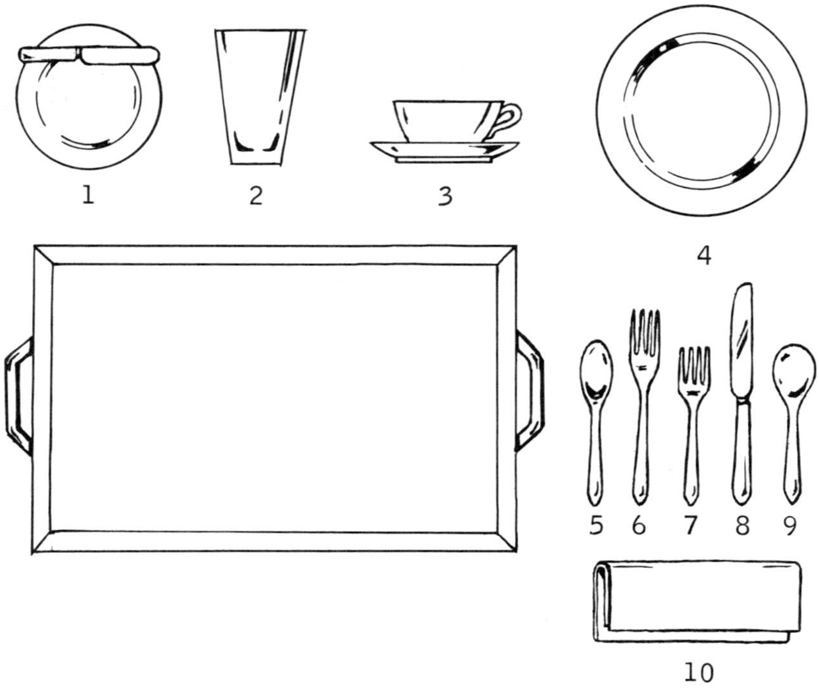

Fig. 19. Serving tray.

3. Match the type of milk with the correct description.

Milk		Description
a. Homogenized	_____ 1.	Heated to specific temperature to remove all harmful bacteria
b. Skim	_____ 2.	Milk left after fat has been removed in making butter
c. Buttermilk	_____ 3.	Whole milk with the fat evenly distributed throughout
d. Pasteurized	_____ 4.	Milk to which 400 I. U. of vitamin D per quart is added
e. Irradiated	_____ 5.	Milk without milk fat

4. Multiple Choice. Circle the number preceding the correct answer. Each question has only one correct answer.

A. Milk is a good source of

(1) Iron, calcium and phosphorus.
(2) Vitamins A and D and iron.
(3) Vitamin A and calcium.

B. Drinking raw milk is harmful because

(1) All bacteria present in milk are disease-producing.
(2) It is harder to digest.
(3) One cannot be certain that the animal from which it came or the persons who handled it were free from disease.

C. Coffee contains the stimulant

(1) Caffeine.
(2) Theobromine.
(3) Tannin.

D. Coffee and tea contain the nutrients

(1) Vitamins A and C.
(2) Minerals and carbohydrates.
(3) None.

E. Citrus fruits are particularly useful as an abundant supply of

(1) Protein.
(2) Carbohydrates.
(3) Vitamin C.

F. The preparation of meat by first browning it in a small amount of fat, then cooking it in liquid, is called

(1) Braising.
(2) Roasting.
(3) Broiling.

G. Puréeing is done by

(1) Putting the food through a sieve.
(2) Mashing the food with a fork or potato masher.
(3) Cutting the food in small pieces.

H. Cocoa and chocolate should be boiled because

(1) It improves the flavor.
(2) It makes them more digestible.
(3) It removes the fat content.

I. When an egg is not fresh

(1) The protein content is greatly reduced.
(2) The white becomes more liquid.
(3) It must be cooked longer for digestibility.

J. Rules for planning and serving meals in a hospital are

(1) Entirely different from those in the home.
(2) Basically the same as those applied in the home.
(3) Not important to the practical nurse.

K. Water used in cooking vegetables should be saved for making soups and gravies because

(1) The water contains food nutrients.
(2) This will improve the flavor.
(3) It helps to keep the water bill at a minimum.

L. Milk should be stored at a temperature of

(1) 32 degrees Fahrenheit.
(2) 38 degrees Fahrenheit.
(3) 50 degrees Fahrenheit.

M. Proper refrigeration not only prevents milk from souring, but it also

(1) Makes milk more digestible.
(2) Preserves the nutrient content.
(3) Improves the nutrient content.

N. The part of cereal grains which is the best source of protein and vitamin B complex is the

(1) Bran or outer layer.
(2) Endosperm or white part.
(3) Germ or heart of grain.

O. In selecting a cereal which is superior in nutritive quality, one would choose

(1) A cooked cereal.
(2) An uncooked cereal.
(3) A whole grain cereal, cooked or uncooked.

P. The protein in cereals is

(1) A complete protein.
(2) An incomplete protein.

Q. The protein in milk is

(1) A complete protein.
(2) An incomplete protein.

R. The acid in most fruits

(1) Has an acid effect on the body.
(2) Has an alkaline effect on the body.

S. Meat is especially necessary in the diet because of

(1) Its high protein content.
(2) Its high carbohydrate content.
(3) Its high fat content.

T. The grades of meat most commonly found in a supermarket are

(1) Prime and choice.
(2) Choice and good.
(3) Good and standard.

5. List several reasons why breakfast should never be omitted.

6. Place a check mark in front of each statement which is an important factor in properly selecting and preparing vegetables in order to obtain the best nutritive value.

____ A. Always use frozen vegetables.
____ B. Wilted and overripe vegetables have less nutritive value.
____ C. Peel them as thinly as possible or cook with skins on.
____ D. Use large quantities of water in cooking.
____ E. Cook them in large pieces.

7. Which vitamins are fat soluble? Which are water soluble?

8. Place a check mark in front of the statements which are considered food fallacies.

____ A. Milk is constipating.
____ B. Onions kill a cold.
____ C. Beets build blood.
____ D. Never mix milk and fish.
____ E. Rare-cooked meat is undigestible.
____ F. Soda makes cabbage digestible.
____ G. One who is trying to lose weight must not drink water.
____ H. Blackstrap molasses cures anemia.
____ I. Skim milk has little nutritive value.
____ J. Toasted bread has fewer calories than fresh bread.

9. From the following list of foods, plan a dinner menu that is nutritive and economical.

Appetizers	Salads
Canned tomato juice	Lettuce and tomato
Frozen orange juice	Fresh citrus fruit
Fresh fruit cup	Gelatin vegetable salad
Canned vegetable soup	Avocado on lettuce
Frozen shrimp	Cole slaw

Main Course
Prime rib roast, potatoes, string beans
Hamburg steaks, noodles, spinach
Macaroni and cheese
Pork chops, apple sauce, peas
Veal cutlet, potatoes, broccoli
Lamb stew

Breads
Hot rolls
Bran muffins
Whole wheat bread
White bread
Cinnamon buns

Beverages
Hot chocolate
Coffee or tea
Milk
Eggnog

Desserts
Canned peaches
Gelatin
Rice pudding
Fruit pie
Cookies and ice cream

Chapter 24

DIET THERAPY

REFERENCES

Culver, V.: Modern Bedside Nursing, Chapter 26.
Hoffman, C., Lipkin, G., and Thompson, E.: Simplified Nursing, Chapter 19.
Howe, P. S.: Nutrition for Practical Nurses, Section II.
Mowry, L.: Basic Nutrition and Diet Therapy for Nurses, Part II.
Rapier, D. K., et al.: Practical Nursing, Chapter 37.
Shackelton, A. D.: Practical Nurse Nutrition Education, Section 2.
Thompson, E., and Murphy, C.: Textbook of Basic Nursing, Chapter 23.

1. Make a complete sentence using each of the following words:

   A. Diet therapy

   B. Modification

   C. Consistency

2. Match the classifications of diets with the types of diet.

Classification		Type
a. Modification according to consistency	____	1. Liquid
b. Modification according to energy value	____	2. High vitamin
c. Modification according to nutrient value	____	3. Low sodium
	____	4. High calorie
	____	5. Soft
	____	6. Bland
	____	7. Low purine
	____	8. Full
	____	9. High protein
	____	10. Low residue

3. Plan a breakfast menu for a full liquid diet.

4. Circle the letters in front of the following foods which may be served in a soft diet.

A. Coffee
B. Mashed potato
C. Broiled steak
D. Chicken rice soup
E. Purêed peas
F. Canned peach halves
G. Eggnog
H. Macaroni and cheese
I. Broiled fish
J. Toast and butter

5. What is meant by the term "a 3 per cent vegetable"?

6. Plan a breakfast menu using 35 grams carbohydrates, 13 grams proteins and 15 grams fats. How many calories does this meal contain?

7. Match each special diet with the disease condition for which it is commonly used.

Special Diet		Disease Condition
a. Low fat	_____	1. Gastric ulcer
b. High protein	_____	2. Atonic constipation
c. Sippy	_____	3. Gallbladder disease
d. Low salt	_____	4. Long-term illnesses and infectious diseases
e. High residue	_____	5. Cardiac disease

8. Match each special diet with the correct description.

Special Diet		Description
a. High caloric	_____	1. Increased amount of roughage
b. High residue	_____	2. Begin with milk and cream and gradually add non-irritating foods in small amounts
c. Low sodium	_____	3. Over four thousand calories daily
d. Sippy	_____	4. Foods prepared without salt

PART V

BASIC NURSING PROCEDURES

Chapter 25

THE PATIENT'S ENVIRONMENT

THE PATIENT'S UNIT
HOUSEKEEPING
BEDMAKING

REFERENCES

Culver, V.: Modern Bedside Nursing, Chapter 33.
Hoffman, C., Lipkin, G., and Thompson, E.: Simplified Nursing, Chapter 20.
Rapier, D. K., et al.: Practical Nursing, Chapters 15, 16 and 19.
Rasmussen, S.: Foundations of Practical and Vocational Nursing, Chapters 5-6.
Thompson, E., and Murphy, C.: Textbook of Basic Nursing, Chapter 25.

THE PATIENT'S UNIT

1. Complete.

   A. The temperature of the patient's room should be______ to______degrees Fahrenheit or______ to ______ degrees Centigrade.

   B. For an ________________ patient, it may be necessary to slightly increase the temperature of the room.

   C. The humidity of the room should be ______ per cent.

   D. A high humidity is sometimes used therapeutically for ____________________ ________________________________.

   E. Ventilation is the process of supplying the ________________ quantity of _______ in the room. In order for a room to have good cross ventilation, there should be windows on ___________ sides and not ____________ one another.

F. As air circulates, ____________ air rises and ____________ air goes to the bottom of the room.

G. Pure air is composed of ________________ , ________________ and ________________ .

H. Good ventilation is important to a patient because ________________________ ________________________ .

I. Drafts can be avoided by placing a ____________ between the window and the ____________ .

J. Sunlight is important because ________________________ .

K. Basic furniture in a patient unit should include ____________ , ____________ , ____________ and ____________ .

L. The patient should be allowed to keep a few personal belongings in the hospital because ________________________ .

2. Many of the personal habits of the nurse have an effect on the patient's attitude toward his surroundings. How can the nurse govern her own habits to

A. Prevent the patient from becoming disturbed by disagreeable odors?

B. Reduce the amount of unnecessary noise?

HOUSEKEEPING

1. Discuss the proper way of disposing of the following waste materials in both the home and hospital:

   A. Bodily excretions

   B. Cotton balls

   C. Food wastes

   D. Sanitary napkins

   E. Soiled dressings

2. List some important points in the care of flowers.

3. Why are insects such as flies or mosquitoes a menace to health?

4. What action should the practical nurse take if she discovers bedbugs

   A. In the hospital?

   B. In the home?

5. What are important factors in the care of each of the following types of equipment?

   A. Glassware

   B. Metalware

   C. Plasticware

   D. Rubber gloves

   E. Wheel chair

6. What should be done with torn linen?

7. Explain how the following stains can be removed from linens:

A. Iodine

B. Blood

C. Grease

D. Coffee or tea

E. Mucus or pus

8. How often should each of the following duties be performed either in the hospital or the home?

A. Thoroughly clean refrigerator

B. Wash bathtub

C. Clean utility room

D. Polish brass and silver

E. Boil patient's utensils

BEDMAKING

1. List the purposes of each of the following articles:

   A. Bath blanket

   B. Rubber draw sheet

   C. Face towel

2. Number the following steps in making an occupied bed in the order in which they should occur:

______ Remove pillows.

______ Loosen all bedding, remove top covers and replace with bath blanket.

______ Make bottom of bed with patient turned first on one side then the other.

______ Replace pillows.

______ Assemble equipment and take to bedside.

______ Remove bath blanket and make top of bed.

3. Discuss the importance of correct bedmaking

   A. To the patient

   B. To the nurse

4. What is meant by the term "open" bed?

5. List three ways in which safety can be observed when making an occupied bed.

6. Multiple Choice. Circle the number preceding the correct answer. There is only one correct answer to each question.

A. A backrest and knee roll may be improvised in the home to take the place of the hospital

(1) Bradford frame.
(2) Balkan frame.
(3) Gatch frame.

B. The simplest method of relieving pressure on the toes from tight bedclothes is to

(1) Use a bed cradle.
(2) Make a toe pleat in the top sheet.
(3) Pull the top bedding over the foot end of the bed.

C. If a pillowcase is too wide for the pillow,

(1) Fold a tuck in one side of the pillowcase.
(2) Try to find a pillowcase that fits.
(3) Send it to the sewing room to be made smaller.

D. The nurse should use good body mechanics while making a bed to

(1) Impress the patient.
(2) Afford the utmost comfort to the patient.
(3) Prevent strain on her own body.

E. When turning a mattress, turn from

(1) Side to side.
(2) Top to bottom.
(3) Side to side and top to bottom.

F. If a patient is allergic to feathers and a nonallergic pillow is not available,

(1) Don't allow the patient to have a pillow.
(2) Cover the pillow with a rubber pillowcase.
(3) Cover the pillow with two cotton pillowcases.

G. Blankets, in order to be both light and warm, should contain

(1) 100 per cent wool.
(2) 25 per cent wool and 75 per cent cotton.
(3) 80 per cent wool and 20 per cent cotton.

H. The top sheet should be turned down over the blanket

(1) 3 inches.
(2) 6 inches.
(3) 9 inches.

I. Hospital spreads are usually made of

(1) Crinkled cotton crepe.
(2) Chenille.
(3) Taffeta.

J. Draw sheets are usually made of

(1) Ticking.
(2) Crinkled cotton crepe.
(3) Muslin.

Chapter 26

THE PATIENT'S COMFORT

CHANGING BODY POSITIONS
PERSONAL HYGIENE
MEETING EMOTIONAL AND SPIRITUAL NEEDS

REFERENCES

Culver, V.: Modern Bedside Nursing, Chapters 32, 35 and 36.
Hoffman, C., Lipkin, G., and Thompson, E.: Simplified Nursing, Chapter 21.
Rapier, D. K., et al.: Practical Nursing, Chapters 18 and 20.
Rasmussen, S.: Foundations of Practical and Vocational Nursing, Chapters 13-15.
Thompson, E., and Murphy, C.: Textbook of Basic Nursing, pp. 263-291.

JOURNALS

Fiore, Mary and Ramphal, Marjorie M.: Prevention of decubitus ulcers. Bedside Nurse, 1:13, Sept.-Oct. 1968.
Flotation therapy. J. Practical Nursing, 19:29, Feb. 1969.

CHANGING BODY POSITIONS

1. Complete.

   A. Good posture for the patient is the ____________'s responsibility.

   B. If a patient is unable to move, he should be assisted to move at least every ________________________________.

   C. If a helpless patient is very heavy, always ____________________ when lifting.

   D. Having the patient sit on the bed with the legs hanging over the edge is called ________________________.

   E. Home devices which may be substituted for a back rest are _______________, ____ and ______________________.

   F. A rubber ring should be covered with a _________________ before placing it under the patient.

   G. Before elevating any part of the patient's body you must first _______________ ____.

   H. Changing the patient's position is important to prevent ____________________, relieve _____________________, ______________________ circulation, and give treatments.

   I. The nurse should always practice good body mechanics when performing duties because ____ ____________.

   J. The main pressure areas of the body are _________________, ____________, ______________________, ______________________ and __________________.

2. On Figure 20 place red under the areas that need support when the patient is resting in each position.

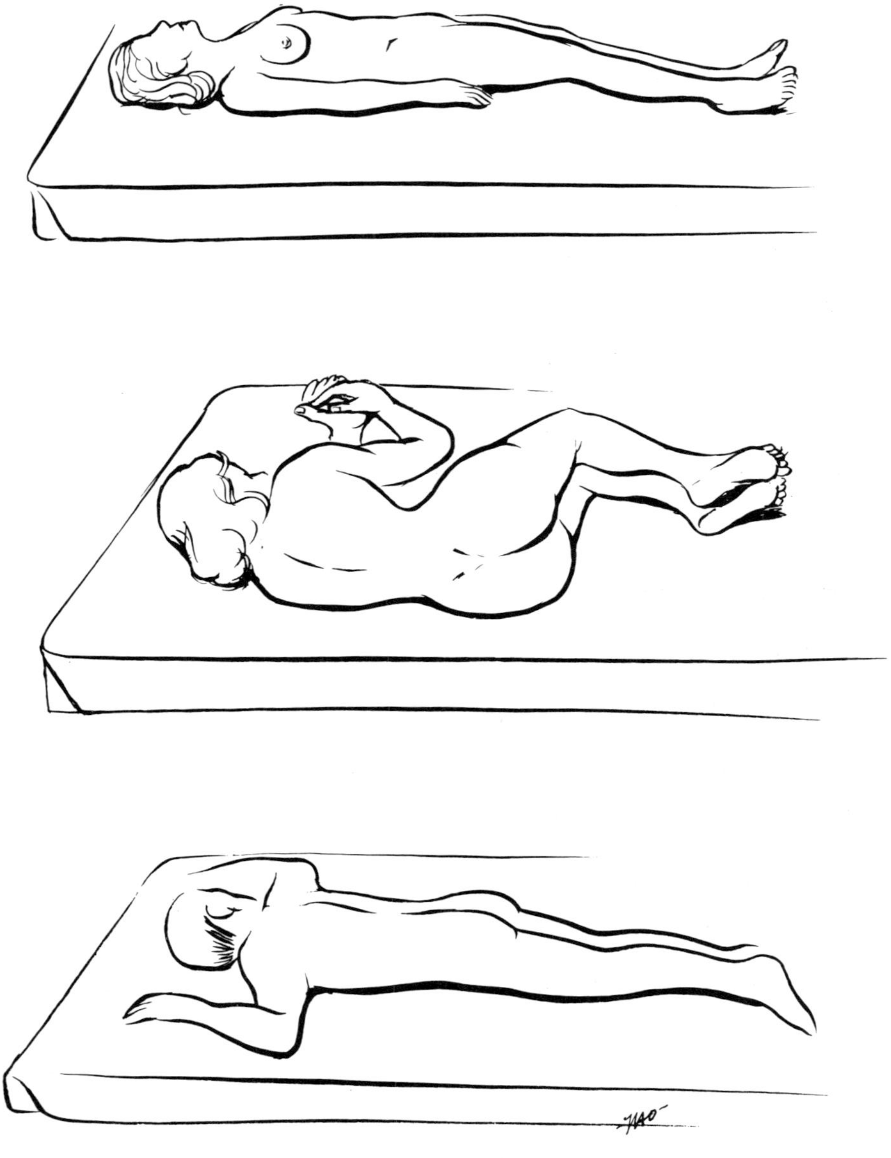

Fig. 20. Positions to aid the patient's comfort.

3. Explain why Figures 21, 22, 23 and 24 picture poor body mechanics on the part of the nurse.

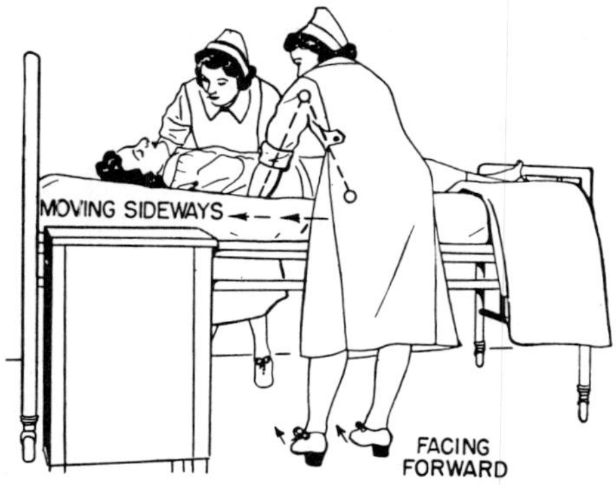

Fig. 21. Poor body mechanics in moving the patient up in bed.

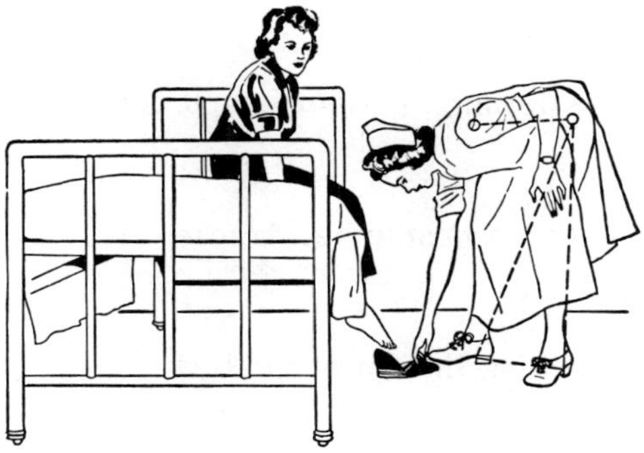

Fig. 22. Poor body mechanics in picking up an object from the floor.

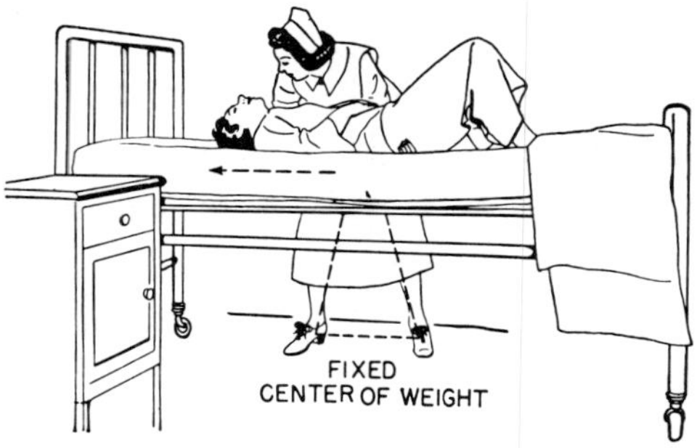

Fig. 23. Poor body mechanics in assisting the patient to move up in bed.

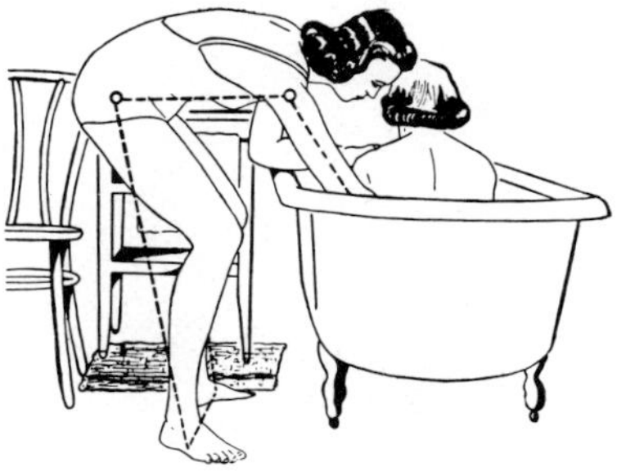

Fig. 24. Poor body mechanics in assisting the patient with a tub bath.

(Illustrations from Fash, Bernice: Body Mechanics in Nursing Arts. New York, McGraw-Hill Book Co., Inc., 1946.)

4. Discuss the treatment of a decubitus ulcer.

5. What are the disadvantages of using "doughnuts" or air rings?

6. List the safety measures which must be used when doing each of the following procedures:

A. Assisting a patient in and out of a wheel chair

B. Using a heated bed cradle

C. Turning the patient in bed

7. Match each device with its purpose.

Device		Purpose
a. Footboard	c.	1. To keep the bedclothes from touching the body
b. Sandbag	d.	2. To protect the patient from falling out of bed.
c. Bed cradle	e.	3. Adjustable, to change the patient's position.
d. Bed sides	a.	4. To prevent footdrop.
e. Gatch bed	b.	5. To immobilize part of the body

PERSONAL HYGIENE

1. What is meant by "total nursing care"?

2. List the duties of the practical nurse involved in

   A. Morning care

   B. Afternoon care

3. What circumstances may necessitate the nurse's using special mouth care?

4. List the safety measures to be remembered when doing each of the following procedures:

   A. Shaving a male patient

   B. Caring for the nails

   C. Giving a bed bath

   D. Giving a shampoo to a bed patient

   E. Giving a tub bath

5. When may it be necessary for the nurse to shave a male patient?

6. How can the nurse help to relieve the patient of embarrassment when giving a complete bath?

7. List the ways in which the nurse can teach the patient good health habits.

8. What solutions may be used as a mouthwash?

9. Define incontinence.

10. List two purposes of each procedure.

  A. Back rub

  B. Cleansing bath

  C. Mouth care

  D. Partial bed bath

11. Complete.

  A. Alcohol used in giving a back rub may be warmed by ____________________

  ____.

  B. The alcohol used for a back rub is a _______ per cent solution.

  C. When giving a bed bath, the water should be changed after washing the

  ________________________.

  D. Fingernails are cared for immediately after ____________________________.

  E. During the bed bath for most patients, the position of the backrest is

  ______________________________.

  F. The temperature of the water for a tub bath should be _________ degrees Fahrenheit.

  G. Pediculi are of two types: ___________ lice and ___________ lice. These insects are obtained from ____.

  H. The treatment of head lice consists of ______________, to kill the insects, and _________________, to kill the nits, or _________________, to kill both.

  I. When the nurse discovers pediculi on a patient, her first step is ___________

  ____.

  J. When removing dentures, place them immediately in a ____________________ and label correctly.

MEETING EMOTIONAL AND SPIRITUAL NEEDS

1. True or False. Circle T if the statement is true; F is the statement is false.

T F 1. A nurse should insist that her patient read good literature.
T F 2. Diversion means anything that diverts the patient's mind from his illness.
T F 3. A long range plan of diversion is more difficult than a short one.
T F 4. Occupations are planned, purposeful activities.
T F 5. Diversional therapy is intended primarily for the aged.
T F 6. A nurse should engage her patient in only those diversional activities she enjoys.
T F 7. What is work for one patient may be play for another.
T F 8. A nurse who encourages her patient to have frequent talks with a clergyman is contributing much to the patient's general welfare.
T F 9. The request for spiritual care should come from the patient.
T F 10. The nurse is required to comply with a patient's religious requests only if the patient has the same religious beliefs as the nurse.
T F 11. Before receiving Holy Communion, the Catholic patient fasts for 3 hours. Water is allowed during this time.
T F 12. Extreme Unction is a sacrament of the Catholic faith and is offered only to the dying patient.
T F 13. In the event of an emergency, the nurse can baptize a patient.
T F 14. Baptism and communion are sacraments of most Protestant faiths.
T F 15. There are no definite rituals that a Jewish patient must engage in prior to surgery or radical therapy.

2. How should the nurse prepare the Catholic patient's unit for Holy Communion?

3. Make a list of rules which you think should apply to discussions about religion with the patient.

Chapter 27

OBSERVING AND RECORDING

CARDINAL SYMPTOMS
COLLECTING SPECIMENS
CHARTING
ADMISSION, TRANSFER AND DISCHARGE
PHYSICAL EXAMINATIONS
POSITIONING AND DRAPING

How well do you observe? As you know, each nurse must learn to be a good observer. It takes a great deal of training and practice for a nurse to become an expert at observing her patient's condition, but here is a little fun exercise to see how well you observe things in general. Allow yourself about one minute to observe Figure 25 carefully, then write a brief paragraph describing what you saw. When you have completed that, do the same with Figures 26 and 27. As you can see, the drawings are not related to nursing.

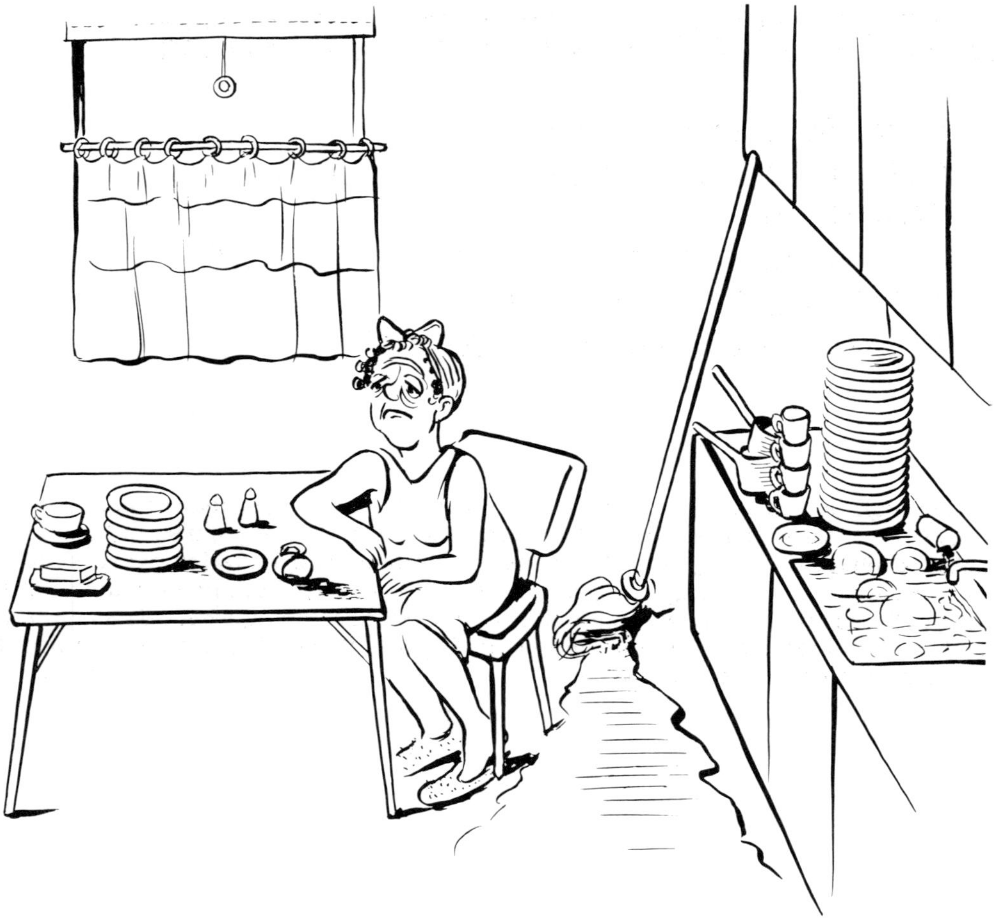

Fig. 25. A sketch to observe.

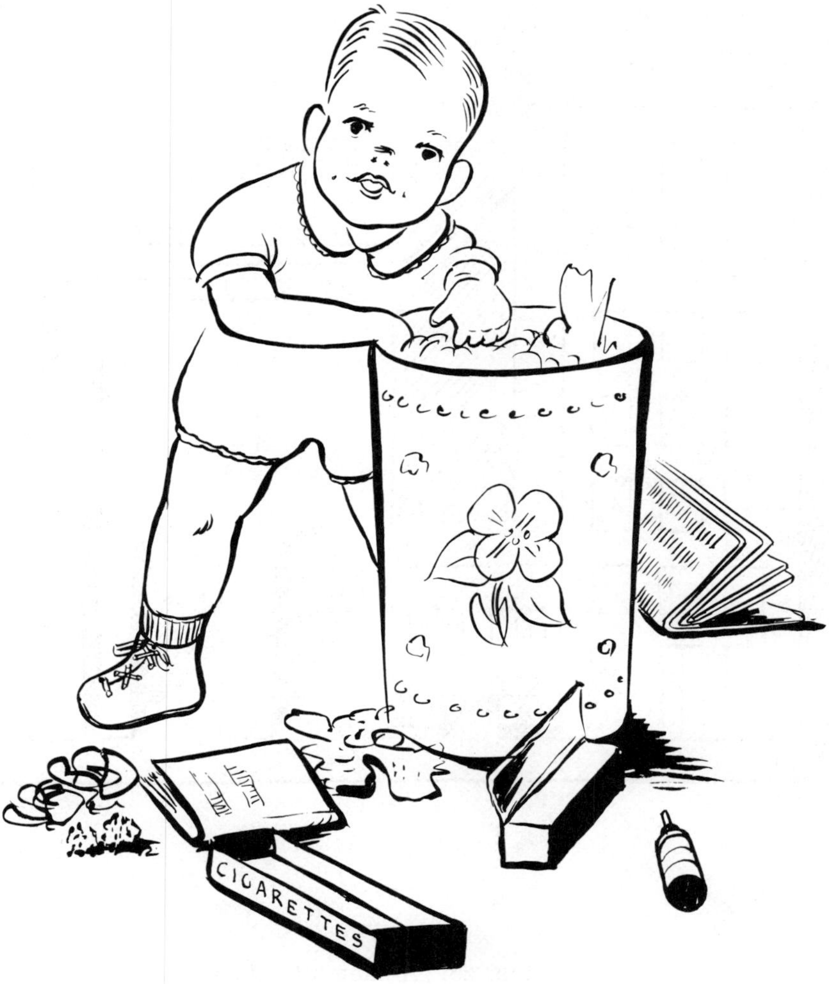

Fig. 26. A sketch to observe.

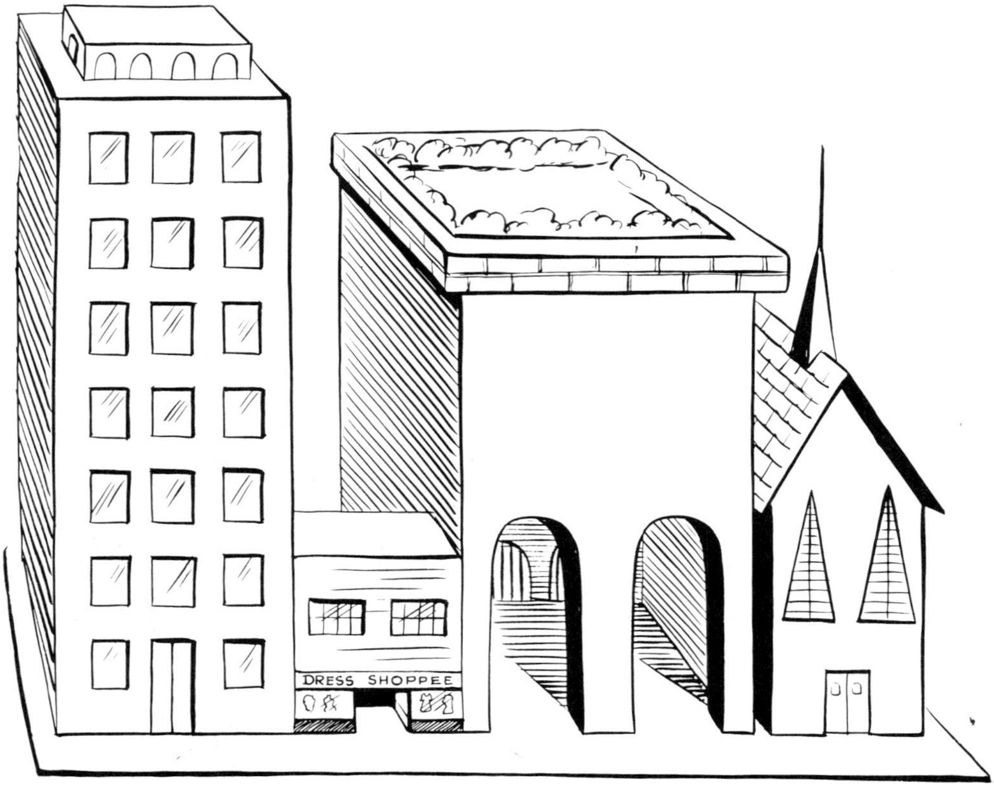

Fig. 27. A sketch to observe.

CARDINAL SYMPTOMS

REFERENCES

Culver, V.: Modern Bedside Nursing, Chapter 34.
Hoffman, C., Lipkin, G., and Thompson, E.: Simplified Nursing, pp. 259-270.
Rapier, D. K., et al.: Practical Nursing, Chapter 22.
Rasmussen, S.: Foundations of Practical and Vocational Nursing, pp. 89-94.
Thompson, E., and Murphy, C.: Textbook of Basic Nursing, pp. 314-324.

THE TEMPERATURE

1. Complete.

A. The normal body temperature is 98.6° degrees Fahrenheit or 37°C degrees Centigrade.

B. Heat in the body is produced by food and muscular activity.

C. The symptoms of an elevated temperature are dry hot, flushed skin and ________.

D. Disturbances which may cause the temperature to rise are infections, dehydration, exercise and ________.

E. Crisis is a sudden fall in temperature.

F. Before taking the temperature, shake the mercury in the thermometer down to at least 94° degrees.

G. Never take a temperature by mouth if the pt is unconscious.

H. The temperature is taken rectally if the pt is unconscious.

I. When taking a rectal temperature, lubricate the bulb, insert the thermometer in the rectum 1 1/2 inches and hold it in place 5 minutes.

J. The temperature is taken by axilla if ________.

K. If you are not certain about the reading of the thermometer, you will take it again with another thermometer.

L. After use, thermometers are washed with ____________________

and stored in ____________________.

2. Practice.

A. Place the correct Fahrenheit reading in the space provided below each thermometer scale shown in Figure 28.

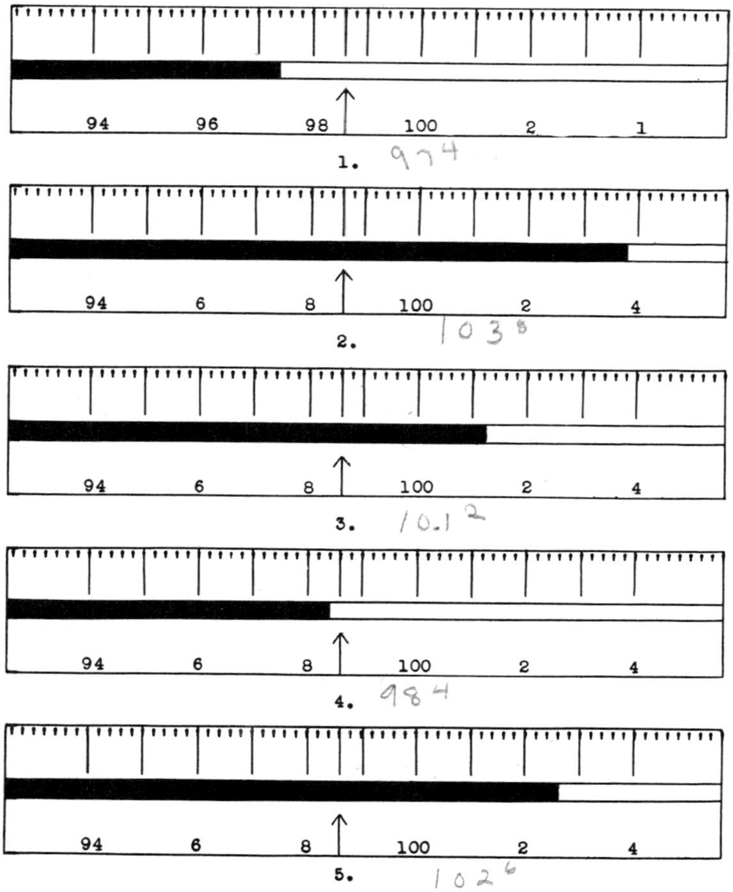

Fig. 28. Thermometer scales.

B. Take the temperatures of five of your classmates and record the correct readings in the space provided.

(1) ____________________

(2) ____________________

(3) ____________________

(4) ____________________

(5) ____________________

THE PULSE

1. Match each word with its definition.

Words		Definition
a. Pulse	g.	1. Number of pulse beats per minute
b. Rhythm	d	2. Pulse rate above 160 per minute
c. Digitalis	f.	3. Strength of the heart beat felt by the fingers
d. Tachycardia	h.	4. Abnormality of volume: weak and running pulse
e. Bradycardia	a	5. The beat which is felt by the blood forced through the arteries
f. Volume	c	6. A drug which slows the pulse rate
g. Rate	b.	7. The spacing of pulse beats
h. Thready	e.	8. A very slow pulse rate
i. Intermittent	j.	9. The artery most frequently used for taking the pulse
j. Radial	I.	10. A pulse beat is skipped at intervals

2. Practice.

A. Take and record the pulse rate of several classmates.
B. Select a partner among your classmates and take her pulse

(1) While she is sitting

(2) After she has walked around for a few minutes

(3) After she has walked up and down the stairs

RESPIRATIONS

1. Multiple Choice. Circle the number preceding the correct answer to each question.

A. Respiration is the mechanism of

(1) Body metabolism.
(2) Exchange of gases in the body.
(3) A disturbed physical condition.

B. The average adult rate of respiration per minute is

(1) 12 to 16.
(2) 16 to 20.
(3) 20 to 30.

C. The rate of respiration may be normally increased by

(1) Sleep.
(2) Fatigue.
(3) Exercise.

D. When taking the respiration,

(1) It is best to perform the procedure unknown to the patient.
(2) Always explain the procedure to the patient.

E. Difficult breathing is called

(1) Apnea.
(2) Dicrotic.
(3) Dyspnea.

F. Abnormal respirations in which there is a cycle beginning with slow, shallow respirations and gradually becoming deep and rapid, then stopping briefly, are called

(1) Orthopnea.
(2) Cheyne-Stokes.
(3) Kussmaul.

G. When counting the rate of respiration,

(1) Count the movements of inspiration and expiration as one.
(2) Count each movement of inspiration and expiration separately.
(3) Count only the movements of inspiration.

H. Practical Nurse E. checked the respirations on a six-month-old infant and noted the rate to be 30 per minute. She should

(1) Report it immediately to the head nurse.
(2) Recheck the rate and report it to the nurse in charge of her nursing team.
(3) Record it and say nothing concerning the rate.

I. One sign of an insufficient amount of oxygen in the body may be

(1) Edema.
(2) Cyanosis.
(3) Crisis.

J. When taking respirations, count for

(1) 15 seconds.
(2) 30 seconds.
(3) 1 minute.

2. Practice.

A. Take and record the respirations of several classmates.

B. Properly record the following temperature, pulse and respiration rates on the sample graphic sheet.

3-1-64:	8:00 A.M.	99.2°	86	18
	4:00 P.M.	99.8°	90	20
	8:00 P.M.	98.4°	84	18
	12:00 P.M.	98°	76	16
3-2-64:	8:00 A.M.	97.6°	74	18
	10:00 A.M.	101.4°	100	22
	4:00 P.M.	103.2°	112	24
	8:00 P.M.	104.6°	120	26
	12:00 P.M.	104.2° (rectally)	116	22
	4:00 A.M.	102.8° (rectally)	110	20
3-3-64:	8:00 A.M.	100.8°	120	26
	12:00 A.M.	99.6°	96	20
	4:00 P.M.	99.2°	90	20
	8:00 P.M.	98.0°	80	18
3-4-64:	8:00 A.M.	97.2°	72	16
	4:00 P.M.	98.2°	76	16

BLOOD PRESSURE

1. Define

A. Systolic pressure - the working stage of the heart

B. Diastolic pressure - the resting stage of the heart

C. Blood pressure the measurement of the blood as it is pumped from the heart into the arteries

D. Hypertension - high blood pressure

E. Hypotension - low blood pressure

2. Number each step in taking the blood pressure in the order in which it should be performed.

__2__ Extend patient's arm, palm side up, and wrap cuff around upper arm.

__1__ Assemble equipment and place properly.

__5__ Open valve on air pump and gradually let air escape.

__3__ Place stethoscope in ears and on patient's arm. Pump air into cuff.

__4__ Close valve on air pump.

3. Practice. Take and record the blood pressures of several classmates.

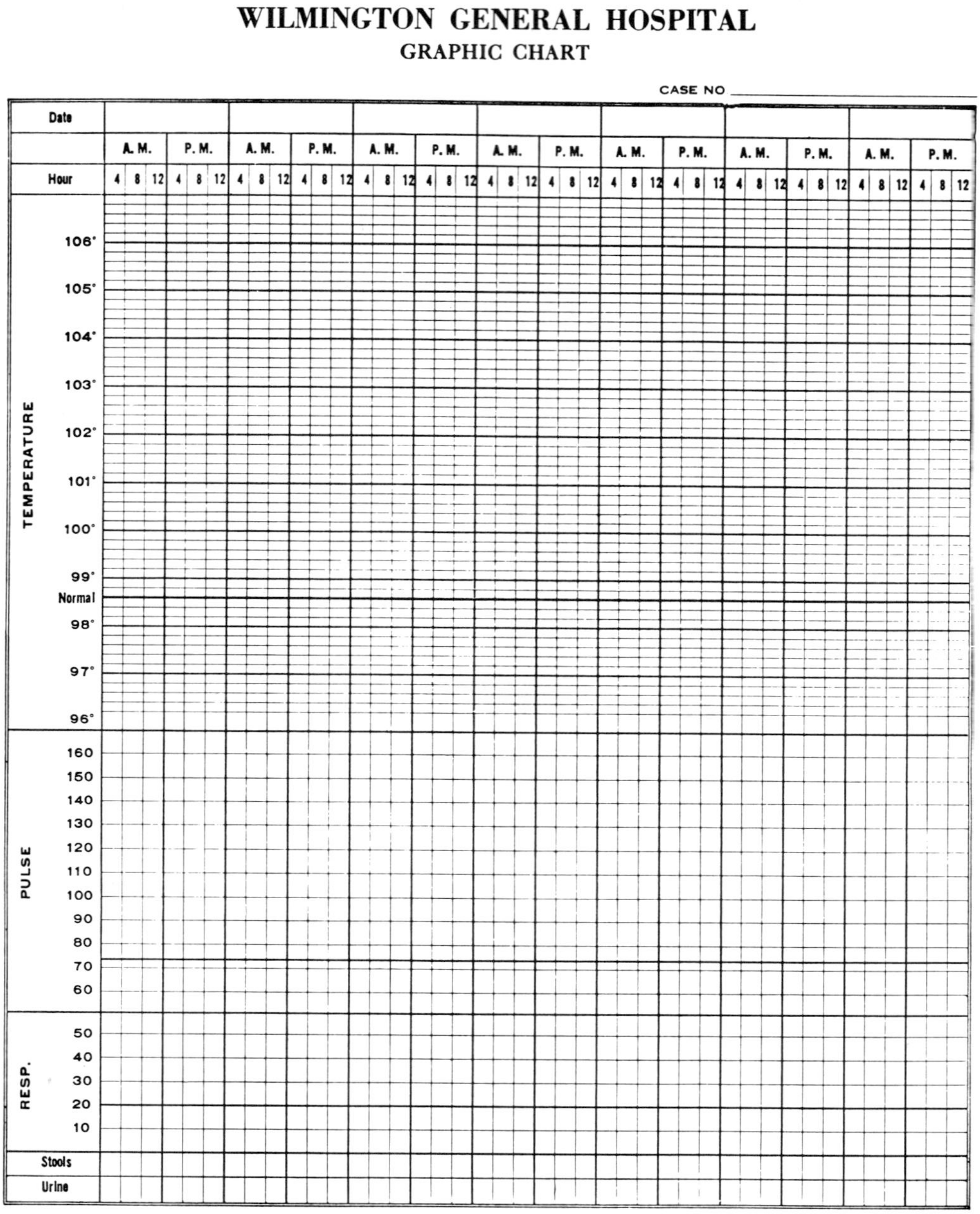

Fig. 29. Sample graphic chart. (Wilmington General Hospital, Wilmington, Delaware.)

COLLECTING SPECIMENS

REFERENCES

Culver, V.: Modern Bedside Nursing, Chapter 34.
Hoffman, C., Lipkin, G., and Thompson, E.: Simplified Nursing, pp. 246-259.
Rapier, D. K., et al.: Practical Nursing, Chapter 24.
Rasmussen, S.: Foundations of Practical and Vocational Nursing, pp. 97-99.
Thompson, E., and Murphy, C.: Textbook of Basic Nursing, Chapter 32.

1. What specimens may be collected in each type of container shown in Figure 30?

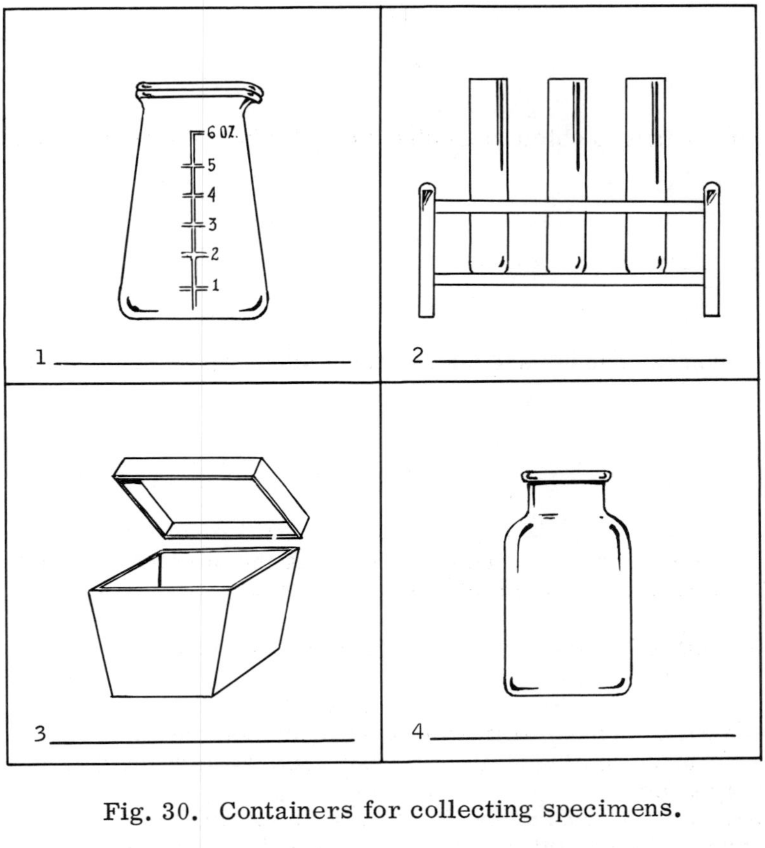

Fig. 30. Containers for collecting specimens.

2. List three abnormal characteristics to be checked in each specimen of

   A. Urine

B. Feces

C. Sputum

D. Vomitus

3. What information should be included in labeling a specimen?

4. Why is it important to obtain specimens exactly how and when specified by the doctor?

5. How many ounces of urine are needed for a single specimen of urine?

6. Multiple Choice. Circle the number preceding the correct answer to each question. There is only one correct answer to each.

A. In collecting a 24-hour urine specimen, an important step in the procedure is to

(1) Keep each voided specimen in a separate container.
(2) Begin the collection at any time but make certain the patient's bladder is empty to start.
(3) Make certain that the specimens are collected only during a time of the day when the patient is not having a bowel movement.

B. In a fractional urinalysis

(1) All urine for a 24-hour period is collected in one specimen bottle.
(2) All urine for a 24-hour period is collected in several bottles labeled for specific time periods.
(3) A dye is first given to the patient, then he is asked to void at intervals.

C. The process of expelling feces is called

(1) Defecation.
(2) Spitting up.
(3) Peristalsis.

D. Vomiting with great force is called

(1) Regurgitation.
(2) Spitting up.
(3) Projectile.

E. If material is expectorated during a cough, the cough is called

(1) Purulent.
(2) Productive.
(3) Infectious.

F. A diagnostic study of the stomach contents is called a

(1) G.I. series.
(2) Gastric analysis.
(3) Fluoroscopy.

G. Before beginning morning care for a patient, the nurse should know whether or not the patient is going to have blood studies because

(1) The patient is not permitted to have a bath prior to some studies.
(2) The practical nurse is responsible for collecting the specimen.
(3) Breakfast is withheld for some studies.

H. When a specimen of spinal fluid is being obtained, the patient

(1) Lies on his side.
(2) Lies on his abdomen.
(3) Sits on the side of the bed.

I. When the nurse is assisting the doctor with a lumbar puncture, an important point for her to remember is that

(1) The procedure is done using a sterile technique.
(2) The procedure causes a great deal of pain.
(3) The patient's hands must be restrained.

J. When a bedridden patient vomits, the nurse can best help the patient by

(1) Immediately calling for help.
(2) Protecting the bed.
(3) Lifting and turning his head to the side.

CHARTING

REFERENCES

Culver, V.: Modern Bedside Nursing, Chapter 34.
Hoffman, C., Lipkin, G., and Thompson, E.: Simplified Nursing, pp. 238-240.
Rapier, D. K., et al.: Practical Nursing.
Rasmussen, S.: Foundations of Practical and Vocational Nursing, pp. 105-127.
Thompson, E., and Murphy, C.: Textbook of Basic Nursing, pp. 409-415.

1. Discuss the uses of the patient's chart.

2. Discuss the meaning of objective and subjective symptoms and give an example of each.

3. Correctly chart the following series of events on the sample bedside notes sheet:

Patient: Mary Jane Smith Room: 415
Diagnosis: Fractured right femur
Orders: Continuous ice bag to right leg
Bed rest
S. S. enema p.r.n.
Full diet
Demerol 100 mg. for pain p.r.n.
Date: 4-15-64

I arrived on duty at 7 A.M. and noticed that Mrs. Smith's call light was on. I went to her room, and she asked me for a bedpan. Fifteen minutes later I collected the pan. She voided 200 cc. At this time she told me that, for a change, she slept well last night. I proceeded to help her wash her hands and face. While doing this, she told me about a good book she is reading. A few minutes after 7:30 her tray was served. She had cooked cereal, scrambled eggs, orange juice, toast and two cups of coffee. It took her about 20 minutes to eat her breakfast, and she ate all her food except a small piece of toast. I also noted that she smoked two cigarettes while drinking her coffee. Around 8 A.M. I started helping her with her bath. She talked a lot during the bath and seemed cheerful today. This is a good improvement because she had been acting very depressed the last few days. I also noticed that she finally got the letter she was expecting from her sister, and I think this is why she is cheerful today. Around 8:30 I gave her a glass of plain tap water to drink (she doesn't like ice water). She sat up in bed to drink it. Around 9:00 A.M. I refilled the ice bag and put a clean cover on it before putting it back on her leg (the right one). At 9:45 her doctor, Dr. Jones, and the head nurse came in to see her. Dr. Jones told the head nurse he wanted Mrs. Smith to have an enema today. The head nurse asked me to give the enema.

I gave her the soapsuds enema around 10 o'clock. Mrs. Smith didn't seem to mind having the enema, and the results were good. After the enema Mrs. Smith spent some time writing letters. A few minutes before 11 she asked for a glass of milk. After she drank the milk, I checked her ice bag, but it didn't need refilling. About 15 minutes before noon, I started getting her ready for lunch. Her ice bag was refilled at this time. She also asked for a bedpan and voided 150 cc. at this time. Lunch was served a few minutes past 12. She ate the sliced chicken, vegetables and salad but would not eat the soup. Shortly after lunch her husband came to visit her. He brought flowers, so I put them in a vase. After Mr. Smith left, I refilled her ice bag and got her fresh water. Before I went off duty at 3, I checked Mrs. Smith, and she was lying on her right side, asleep.

Student Practical Nurse
Lucille Baldwin

WILMINGTON GENERAL HOSPITAL

BEDSIDE NOTES

NAME____________________ MEDICAL NO.____________

DATE	HR.	NOURISHMENT	MEDICATION	REMARKS	URINE	STOOL

Form B-18 — Sterling Printing Co., Wilmington, Del.

Fig. 31. Sample bedside notes sheet. (Wilmington General Hospital, Wilmington, Delaware.)

ADMISSION, TRANSFER AND DISCHARGE

REFERENCES

Culver, V.: Modern Bedside Nursing, Chapter 34.
Hoffman, C., Lipkin, G., and Thompson, E.: Simplified Nursing, pp. 182-189.
Rapier, D. K., et al.: Practical Nursing, Chapter 17.
Rasmussen, S.: Foundations of Practical and Vocational Nursing, pp. 207-208.
Thompson, E., and Murphy, C.: Textbook of Basic Nursing, Chapter 26.

---

1. Complete.

A. When the patient arrives at the hospital, he may have many fears which may be caused by ____

____.

B. The nurse who admits the patient carries an important role in attempting to adjust the patient's mental attitudes. She can fulfill this role by __________

____

____.

C. While admitting the patient, it is the nurse's responsibility to observe ______

____

D. All valuables the patient may bring with him on admission to the hospital should be____.

E. When it is time for the patient to go home, the ____________________ must write an order for the discharge.

F. The attitudes of the nurse toward the patient are just as important upon discharge as upon admission because ______________________________

____.

G. When transferring a patient from one unit to another, articles such as ______________________________ are transferred with the patient.

H. When caring for a patient who insists upon leaving the hospital before the doctor orders the discharge, you should ______________________________

______________________________.

I. When a patient is admitted to the hospital, the ______________________ writes all the directions for the patient's care.

J. When a relative accompanies a patient to the hospital for admission, the nurse can help to ease the relative's anxieties by ______________________

______________________________.

2. You are asked to admit a patient to his room. His name is James Ross. He is brought to the surgical floor at 2 P.M. on a stretcher. You take him to room 312, get him undressed and check his cardinal signs. His T.P.R. is 100-96-20 and B.P. is 120/80. While you are taking his blood pressure, he vomits. You note that the vomitus looks like coffee grounds. The patient tells you that he has a stomach ulcer.

A. What additional procedures will you have to do to complete the admission of this patient?

B. What information regarding the admission will you record on this patient's chart?

PHYSICAL EXAMINATIONS
POSITIONING AND DRAPING

REFERENCES

Culver, V.: Modern Bedside Nursing, Chapters 28 and 34.
Hoffman, C., Lipkin, G., and Thompson, E.: Simplified Nursing, pp. 240-246.
Rapier, D. K., et al.: Practical Nursing, Chapter 23.
Rasmussen, S.: Foundations of Practical and Vocational Nursing, pp. 100-105.
Thompson, E., and Murphy, C.: Textbook of Basic Nursing, pp. 250-255.

1. List five of the nurse's responsibilities in assisting the doctor with a physical examination.

2. Correctly identify and list the purpose of each instrument shown in Figure 32 used by the physician in the physical examination of the patient.

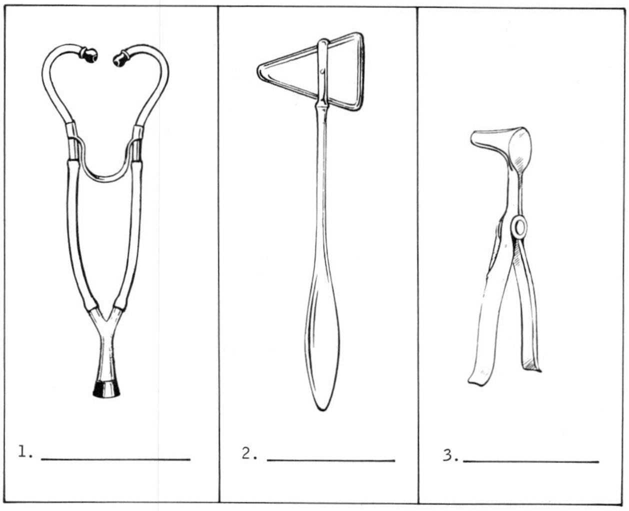

Fig. 32. Instruments used in physical examinations. (Dittmar and Penn Corporation, Philadelphia.)

3. Identify each position of the patient shown in Figure 33 and name one purpose of each position.

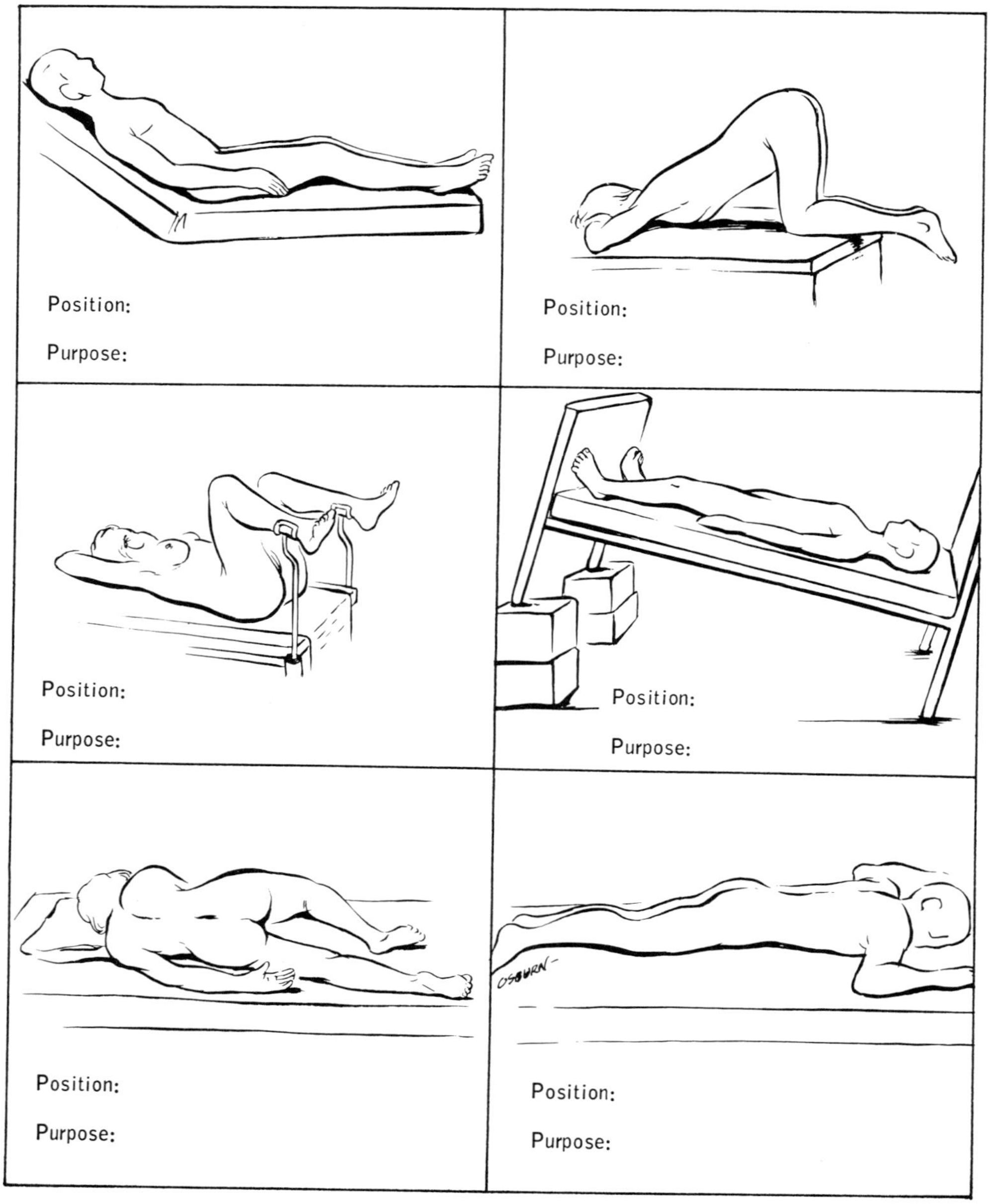

Fig. 33. Positions for the patient.

Chapter 28

THERAPEUTIC SKILLS

THE APPLICATION OF HEAT AND COLD
ENEMAS
IRRIGATIONS
EMERGENCY NURSING
BANDAGING AND BINDERS
PREOPERATIVE AND POSTOPERATIVE NURSING CARE
CARE OF THE DYING AND DEAD

THE APPLICATION OF HEAT AND COLD

REFERENCES

Culver, V.: Modern Bedside Nursing, Chapters 40 and 41.
Hoffman, C., Lipkin, G., and Thompson, E.: Simplified Nursing, pp. 282-293.
Rapier, D. K., et al.: Practical Nursing, pp. 204-206 and Chapter 27.
Rasmussen, S.: Foundations of Practical and Vocational Nursing, pp. 265-275.
Thompson, E., and Murphy, C.: Textbook of Basic Nursing, pp. 292-301.

HEAT

1. List three purposes of applying heat to the body.

2. In what conditions does the physician usually order hot moist applications in preference to hot dry applications?

3. Supply the correct information concerning each treatment.

   A. Applying a hot water bottle

      (1) Temperature of water

      (2) Amount of water to put in bag

      (3) Substitutes for a hot water bottle

   B. Applying hot moist compresses

      (1) Solutions used

      (2) Circumstances under which compresses must remain sterile

      (3) Purpose of applying petroleum jelly to the area to be treated

   C. Sitz bath

      (1) Position of the patient

      (2) Temperature of water

      (3) Information to be charted

D. Oatmeal bath

(1) Purpose

(2) Method of preparing oatmeal

(3) Aftercare of the patient

E. Steam inhalations

(1) Home substitutes

(2) Position of patient

(3) Instructions to the patient

4. Mrs. Jones has an order for the application of a heat lamp to the perineal area for twenty minutes. Ten minutes after you have applied the lamp Mrs. Jones complains that the heat is burning her. What would you do?

5. Place a check mark in front of the equipment needed to give unsterile hot moist dressings.

A. Small basin
B. Large piece of muslin
C. Rubber sheet
D. Face towel
E. Tongue blade or applicators
F. Gauze squares
G. Bulb syringe
H. Petroleum jelly
I. Safety pins
J. Large pitcher
K. Electric plate
L. Kelly pad
M. Two forceps
N. Waste receptacle
O. Solution

COLD

1. List the purposes of applying cold to the body.

2. Supply the correct information concerning each treatment.

A. Applying an ice bag

(1) Safety measures

(2) Aftercare of the bag

B. Cold eye compresses

(1) Position of patient

(2) Precautions

C. Temperature sponge bath

(1) Solutions used

(2) Order of parts to be sponged

(3) When temperature, pulse and respiration should be checked

ENEMAS

REFERENCES

Culver, V.: Modern Bedside Nursing, Chapters 40 and 41.
Hoffman, C., Lipkin, G., and Thompson, E.: Simplified Nursing, pp. 294-301.
Rapier, D. K., et al.: Practical Nursing, pp. 182-188.
Rasmussen, S.: Foundations of Practical and Vocational Nursing, Chapter 22.
Thompson, E., and Murphy, C.: Textbook of Basic Nursing, pp. 302-308.

1. Complete.

   A. An enema is an injection of ______________ into the ____________________ for the purpose of ____.

   B. No enema should be given unless the physician ______________________ ____________________________.

   C. Taking enemas habitually is ______________________________________ because ____.

   D. In giving a cleansing enema, enough solution must be injected into the ______ ______________________________ to __________________________ the feces and ______________________________ peristalsis.

   E. The amount of solution given in a cleansing enema for adults should be ______ __________ to __________ cc.; for children, the amount should be ______ to ___ cc.

   F. When administering an enema, the solution should be prepared at __________ degrees Fahrenheit.

   G. When giving an enema, place the patient in ______________ position because ____.

   H. Never hold the enema can higher than _________ inches above the anus because ____.

I. Before inserting the rectal tube, always ______________ it to prevent discomfort to the patient.

J. If the solution does not flow when giving an enema, the nurse should ______________________________________.

2. Match each type of enema with the correct purpose.

Enema		Purpose
a. Carminative	b	1. Checks diarrhea
b. Emollient	c	2. To soften a hardened fecal mass
c. Oil	a	3. Stimulates the expulsion of flatus from the colon
d. Medicated	d	4. To administer drugs

3. Match each term with the correct definition.

Term		Definition
a. Flatus tube	____	1. Discharge of feces
b. Suppository	____	2. Tube inserted into the rectum for relief of intestinal flatus
c. Fecal impaction	____	3. Removal of enema solution which the patient cannot expel
d. Defecation	____	4. A cone-shaped, medicated object which melts at body temperature
e. Siphonage	____	5. Hardened fecal mass

4. What is the purpose of the retention enema?

5. How long should the retention enema be retained?

6. What is the maximum amount of solution which should be given for the retention enema?

7. List the equipment used in giving a retention enema which differs from that used in giving a nonretention enema.

8. You are administering a cleansing enema to Mrs. Black. You have given her 100 cc. of solution and she begins to complain of abdominal discomfort and states that she cannot retain any more of the solution. What will you do?

IRRIGATIONS

REFERENCES

Culver, V.: Modern Bedside Nursing, Chapters 40 and 41.
Hoffman, C., Lipkin, G., and Thompson, E.: Simplified Nursing, pp. 301, 307.
Rapier, D. K., et al.: Practical Nursing, pp. 187, 193, 199.
Rasmussen, S.: Foundations of Practical and Vocational Nursing, p. 281.
Thompson, E., and Murphy, C.: Textbook of Basic Nursing, pp. 308, 312-313.

---

1. Supply the correct information concerning each type of irrigation.

    A. Colonic irrigation

      (1) Purposes

      (2) Solutions used

      (3) Amount of solution needed

      (4) Length of time needed to administer the irrigation

    B. Colostomy irrigation

      (1) Purposes

      (2) Position of patient

      (3) Amount of solution injected into the colon at one time

    C. Throat irrigation

      (1) Purposes

      (2) Position of patient

      (3) Temperature of solution

    D. Vaginal irrigation

      (1) Purposes

      (2) Contraindications

    E. Eye irrigation

      (1) Position of patient

      (2) Direction of the flow of the solution

2. On the sample bedside notes sheet, correctly record each type of irrigation given. Assume that the expected results were obtained and chart them as such.

A. Colostomy irrigation

B. Colonic irrigation

C. Throat irrigation

D. Eye irrigation

E. Vaginal irrigation

3. Multiple Choice. Circle the number preceding the correct answer to each statement.

A. The colon is lined with

(1) Mucous membrane.

(2) Serous membrane.

(3) Endometrium.

B. The length of the vaginal canal is about

(1) 3 inches.

(2) 6 inches.

(3) 9 inches.

C. An artificial anus is called a

(1) Cystotomy.

(2) Colostomy.

(3) Colectomy.

D. When giving a colonic irrigation, the size rectal tube used is a

(1) Number 16 French.

(2) Number 24 French.

(3) Number 30 French.

E. When giving a throat irrigation, the nozzle should not be allowed to touch the back of the throat in order to prevent

(1) Burning the throat.

(2) The spread of infection.

(3) The patient from gagging.

WILMINGTON GENERAL HOSPITAL

BEDSIDE NOTES

NAME____________________________ MEDICAL NO.________________

DATE	HR.	NOURISHMENT	MEDICATION	REMARKS	URINE	STOOL

Form B-18 — Sterling Printing Co., Wilmington, Del.

Fig. 34. Sample bedside notes sheet. (Wilmington General Hospital, Wilmington, Delaware.)

F. After administering any type of irrigation, the nurse should always

(1) Thoroughly wash her hands.

(2) Explain the procedure to the patient.

(3) Disinfect the equipment.

G. One commercially made colostomy set is named

(1) Binkley.

(2) Cobolt.

(3) Wangensteen.

H. When giving a vaginal irrigation, the nozzle should be rotated to

(1) Prevent air from going through the tube.

(2) Decrease the pressure of the flow.

(3) Insure thorough cleansing.

I. A bulb syringe may be substituted for an irrigating can in performing the

(1) Eye irrigation.

(2) Colonic irrigation.

(3) Vaginal irrigation.

J. The skin around the colostomy stoma should be cleansed with

(1) Sterile saline.

(2) A prescribed ointment.

(3) Soap and water.

EMERGENCY NURSING

REFERENCES

Culver, V.: Modern Bedside Nursing, Chapter 51.
Hoffman, C., Lipkin, G., and Thompson, E.: Simplified Nursing, pp. 509-524.
Rapier, D. K., et al.: Practical Nursing, Chapter 31.
Rasmussen, S.: Foundations of Practical and Vocational Nursing, Chapter 27.
Thompson, E., and Murphy, C.: Textbook of Basic Nursing, pp. 619-633.

---

1. Match each term with the correct definition.

Term		Definition
a. Emergency	_____	1. Nosebleed
b. First aid	_____	2. A break in the skin
c. Wound	_____	3. A condition requiring immediate action
d. Shock	_____	4. Treatment given at the scene of an accident
e. Epistaxis	_____	5. A state of collapse due to circulatory failure
f. Antidote	_____	6. A device used to apply pressure
g. Fracture	_____	7. An artery in the neck
h. Asphyxia	_____	8. A break in a bone
i. Tourniquet	_____	9. An agent for counteracting poison
j. Carotid		

2. Match each emergency condition with the correct treatment.

Condition		Treatment
a. Fainting	_____	1. Immobilize the part
b. Epistaxis	_____	2. Place the victim in a cool place; place him on his back and elevate the head and shoulders
c. Frostbite		
d. Fracture	_____	3. Keep the patient upright, apply cold compresses and pressure to the part
e. Sunstroke		
	_____	4. Never rub the part; place it in cool or lukewarm water
	_____	5. Elevate the lower part of the body

3. Match each emergency condition with the correct symptoms.

Condition		Symptoms
a. Shock	_____	1. The skin is charred and the subcutaneous tissue is destroyed
b. Sunstroke		
c. Third degree burn	_____	2. Abdominal cramps, nausea and vomiting
d. First degree burn	_____	3. Pallor, perspiration, cold extremities and weak, rapid pulse
e. Poisoning		
	_____	4. The skin is reddened
	_____	5. Headache, dizziness, nausea and faintness

4. Match each poison with the correct antidote.

Poison		Antidote
a. Acid	______	1. Diluted vinegar
b. Lye	______	2. Coffee
c. Alcohol	______	3. Coffee and keep the patient active
d. Opiates	______	4. Oxygen and artificial respiration
e. Carbon monoxide	______	5. Baking soda

5. Place a red line across the area where pressure should be applied for the first aid treatment of the external bleeding shown in each section of Figure 37.

6. List five good qualities the emergency nurse should possess.

7. What would be your first three steps of action in each of the following emergency situations? Write them in the order in which you would perform them.

A. A child, in a home in which you are working, pushes a dried bean into his nose.

B. An electrical repairman working in your home touches a live wire.

C. Your neighbor calls you and tells you she was stung by a wasp. She asks your advice.

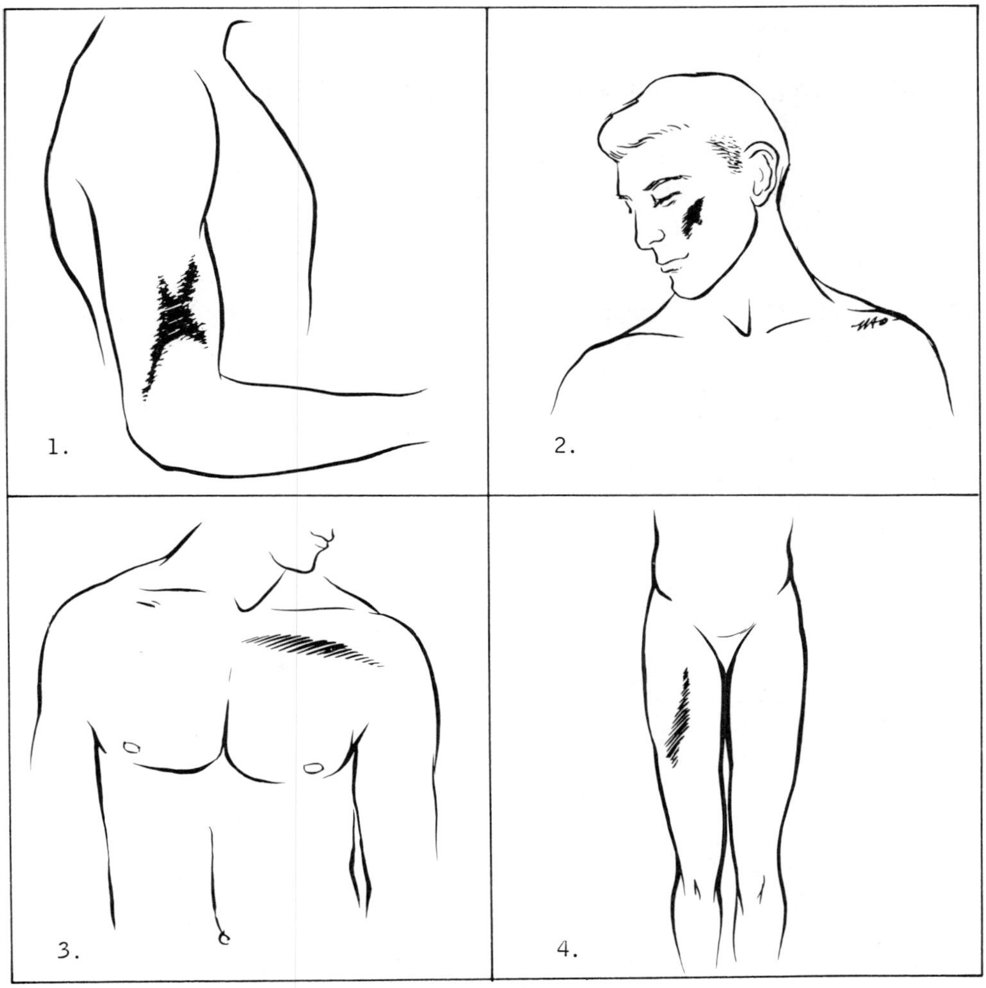

Fig. 35. Areas of external hemorrhage.

D. While you are shopping, you notice a man nearby is beginning to have convulsions.

E. When taking a walk, you see a person lying on the sidewalk.

F. A friend's child falls from a tree. There is a possibility that his arm is fractured.

PREOPERATIVE AND POSTOPERATIVE NURSING CARE

REFERENCES

Culver, V.: Modern Bedside Nursing, Chapter 41.
Hoffman, C., Lipkin, G., and Thompson, E.: Simplified Nursing, Chapter 28.
Keane, C. B.: Essentials of Nursing, 2nd ed. Philadelphia, W. B. Saunders Co., 1969, Chapter 5.
Rapier, D. K., et al.: Practical Nursing, Chapter 30.
Rasmussen, S.: Foundations of Practical and Vocational Nursing, Chapter 25.
Thompson, E., and Murphy, C.: Textbook of Basic Nursing, Chapter 33.

JOURNAL

Argamaso, Ravelo V.: Skin grafts and the care of the grafted patient. Bedside Nurse, 1:11, Nov.-Dec. 1968.

1. What is the purpose of each of the following preoperative orders?

   A. Cleansing enema

   B. "Prep" the surgical site

   C. Nothing by mouth twelve hours prior to surgery

   D. Seconal at bedtime on the evening before surgery

   E. Demerol and atropine to be given one-half hour prior to surgery

2. What is the purpose of each of the following preoperative nursing procedures performed on the morning of surgery?

   A. Removal of dentures

   B. Removal of nail polish

   C. Having the patient void before going to surgery?

3. What is the purpose of the recovery bed?

4. What is the purpose of the recovery room?

5. List the purpose of each of the following postoperative duties of the nurse.

   A. Keeping the patient's head turned to the side

   B. Assisting the patient to move periodically, as ordered

   C. Examining the dressings frequently

6. What are the symptoms of a reaction to a blood transfusion?

7. List the symptoms of each common postoperative complication.

   A. Hemorrhage

   B. Shock

   C. Wound infection

   D. Respiratory difficulty

8. On the sample bedside notes sheet (Figure 36), correctly record the series of preoperative and postoperative events which involved the patient, Mrs. Mary Kay, Room 1001, on her day of surgery for a hemorrhoidectomy.

The patient was awakened early in order to give her an enema at 6:00 A.M., and 100 cc. of warm soapsuds solution was administered into the colon with the patient lying in Sim's position. The results of the enema were good. Breakfast is usually served at 7:30 A.M., but Mrs. Kay has been on nothing by mouth since midnight. We checked her T.P.R. at this time. The readings were 98.6° F., 80, 18. Around 8:15, we started morning care. The patient seemed cheerful and kept up a continual conversation during the procedure. She talked mostly about a book she is reading. After morning care her wedding band was properly secured to her finger and her wrist watch was placed in the safe. At 8:35 a registered nurse came in and gave Mrs. Kay Demerol, 50 mg., and scopolamine, gr. 1/150 I.M. At 9:00 A.M. the patient's husband arrived. Shortly after that we had to ask him to step outside the room so that Mrs. Kay could use the bedpan. She voided two hundred cc. of urine. At 9:30, an operating room attendant arrived for the patient. She was assisted in moving onto a stretcher, and a head covering and operating room stockings were put on her. The attendant then took her to the operating room. We talked briefly to Mr. Kay, then prepared the room for her return.

Mrs. Kay returned to her own room from the recovery room at 12:15 P.M. We moved her from the stretcher to her bed, checked the rectal dressings, tucked in the top bed covers, and checked her blood pressure, pulse and respiration. The readings were 116/76, 92, 20. These were rechecked every half-hour for the next two hours. The readings were: 120/80, 80, 18; 124/82, 88, 18; 118/78, 78, 16; 120/76, 80, 16. At 2:30 P.M. the patient's dressings were reinforced and a clean T binder was applied. There was no bleeding from the operative site. Mrs. Kay was fully awake at this time.

WILMINGTON GENERAL HOSPITAL

BEDSIDE NOTES

NAME ______________________________ MEDICAL NO. ______________

DATE	HR.	NOURISHMENT	MEDICATION	REMARKS	URINE	STOOL

Form B-18 — Sterling Printing Co., Wilmington, Del.

Fig. 36. Sample bedside notes sheet. (Wilmington General Hospital, Wilmington, Delaware.)

9. List the measures which are incorporated to relieve the following in the post-operative care of the patient.

A. Pain

B. Thirst

C. Abdominal distention

D. Retention of urine

E. Constipation

BANDAGING AND BINDERS

REFERENCES

Culver, V.: Modern Bedside Nursing, Chapter 51.
Hoffman, C., Lipkin, G., and Thompson, E.: Simplified Nursing, pp. 525-529.
Rapier, D. K., et al.: Practical Nursing, pp. 142-147.
Rasmussen, S.: Foundations of Practical and Vocational Nursing, pp. 183-188.
Thompson, E., and Murphy, C.: Textbook of Basic Nursing, pp. 633-638.

1. Identify and name the purposes of each fundamental turn used in applying a bandage.

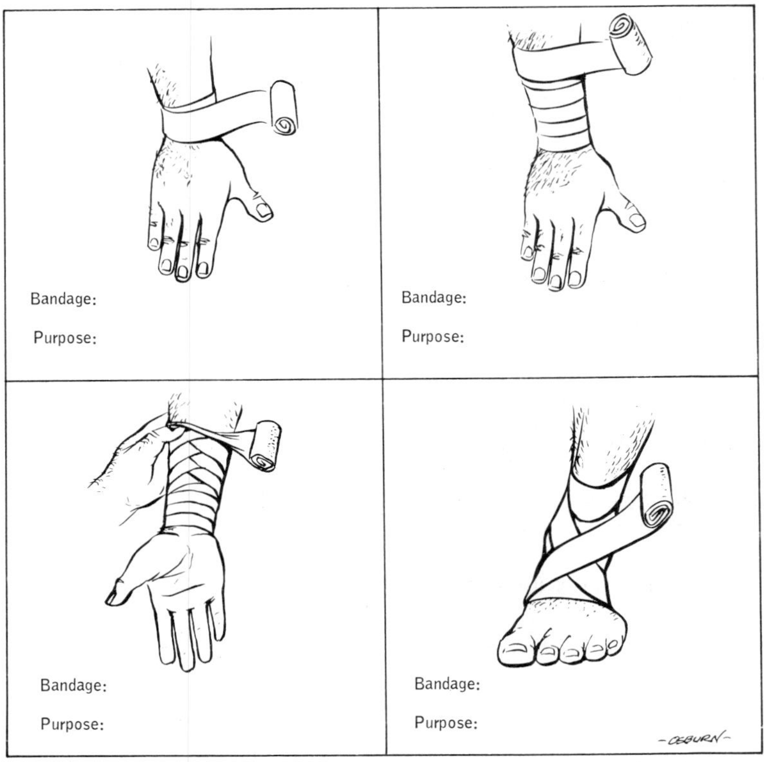

Fig. 37. Turns used in bandaging.

2. Which width bandage would be most appropriate for use in bandaging the following parts of the body?

   A. Fingers

   B. Arm

   C. Chest

3. How can one tell if a bandage has been applied too tightly?

4. How should the ends of the bandage be secured?

5. Describe the uses of the plaster of Paris bandage and explain the method used in applying the bandage.

6. List the three uses of the triangular bandage.

7. What may be used in improvising a

   A. Straight binder?

   B. T binder?

8. Name a solution used to remove adhesive tape from the skin.

9. What precaution is necessary when using this solution?

10. Identify and list the purposes of each type of binder shown in Figure 38.

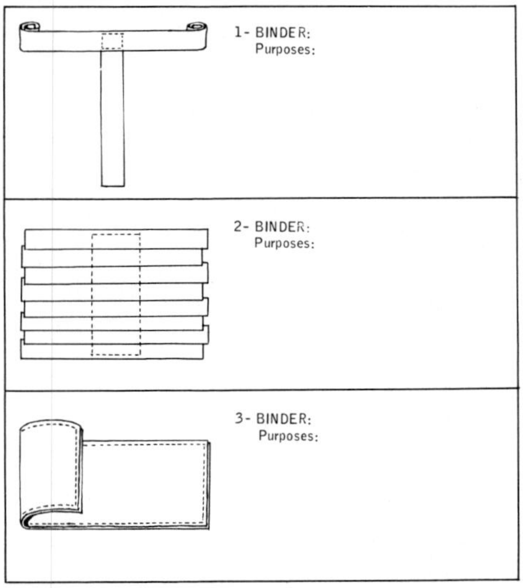

Fig. 38. Types of binders.

CARE OF THE DYING AND DEAD

REFERENCES

Culver, V.: Modern Bedside Nursing, Chapter 39.
Hoffman, C., Lipkin, G., and Thompson, E.: Simplified Nursing, pp. 321-324.
Rapier, D. K., et al.: Practical Nursing, Chapter 32.
Rasmussen, S.: Foundations of Practical and Vocational Nursing, pp. 663-664.

1. Discuss each of the following:

   A. Consider these two critically ill elderly patients. Both have been told by their doctor that they are going to die. Patient A. talks about death to you frequently. He talks about the pleasurable and full life he has lived and states that he knows his life may end any time. In contrast, Patient B. never talks about death; instead he continues to discuss plans for the future. What do you think are the feelings of each of these patients concerning death?

   B. Mrs. X. has not been told that she is going to die. During morning care she asks, "Am I going to die?" You are aware that death is expected in the near future. What answer will you give Mrs. X.?

2. What nursing procedures are necessary for the dying patient

   A. To prevent the mouth from becoming dry?

   B. To relieve breathing difficulties?

3. What provisions are made for the spiritual comfort of the dying patient who is a member of

A. The Catholic faith?

B. The Jewish faith?

4. True or False. Circle T if the statement is true; F if the statement is false. Correct the statements that are false by crossing out the incorrect word or words and writing the correct word or words in the space above.

T F 1. The nurse must decide whether or not the patient should be told he is not going to live.

T F 2. Cheyne-Stokes respirations are common in the dying patient.

T F 3. Hearing is usually the first sense to leave the dying patient.

T F 4. When a patient expires in the home, the first person the nurse should call is the undertaker.

T F 5. If the patient who expires has a private practical nurse, it is the nurse's responsibility to inform the relatives of the patient's death.

T F 6. Dentures must be placed in the patient's mouth as soon as possible after death.

T F 7. After death, the patient's jewelry and other valuables should be properly labeled and sent with the patient to the morgue.

T F 8. The nurse in the home may assist the family at the time of death by insisting that they regularly take sedatives.

T F 9. Regardless of the diagnosis, following a patient's death the unit must be cleaned and disinfected in the same manner as following an infectious disease.

T F 10. The procedure for the care of the body after death is usually alike in all hospitals.

Chapter 29

CONTROLLING DISEASE

MICROBIOLOGY
ASEPTIC TECHNIQUES

Microbiology

MICROORGANISMS

BODY PROTECTION AGAINST DISEASE

METHODS OF DISEASE TRANSMISSION AND CONTROL

REFERENCES

Culver, V.: Modern Bedside Nursing, Chapter 27.
Hoffman, C. P., Lipkin, G. B., and Thompson, E. M.: Simplified Nursing, pp. 16-22.
Keane, C. B.: Essentials of Nursing, Chapter 2.
Rasmussen, S.: Foundations of Practical and Vocational Nursing, Chapter 3.
Thompson, E., and Murphy, C.: Textbook of Basic Nursing, Chapter 7.

---

1. Match Column I with Column II.

Column I		Column II
a. Pathogenic	c	1. Oval-shaped bacteria
b. Bacilli	b	2. Rod-shaped bacteria
c. Cocci	d	3. Spiral-shaped bacteria
d. Spirilla	e	4. Protective covering
e. Spore	a	5. Disease-producing

2. Complete.

Microorganisms feed upon both living and dead substances. They grow best in ____________, ____________, ____________ places. Bacteria are only one type of microorganism. Another type, commonly known, is the ____________, the smallest of microorganisms. The word "germ" is commonly used in discussing the causes of disease. The term "germ" includes ____________ types of microorganisms which cause disease.

3. Multiple Choice. Circle the number preceding the correct answer to each statement.

A. The method of transmission by which disease-producing organisms are transferred through moisture expelled in sneezing is called

(1) Human carrier.
(2) Droplet infection.
(3) Vectors.

B. Substances which the blood forms to neutralize bacterial toxins are

(1) White blood cells.
(2) Toxins.
(3) Antibodies.

C. An immune person

(1) Is free from the risk of specific infections.
(2) Is free from bacteria.
(3) Has an increased amount of white corpuscles in the blood.

D. When one has acquired active immunity, this means

(1) Substances have been injected into the body to stimulate the body to produce antibodies.
(2) Specific antibodies were present in the body at birth.
(3) Antibodies were first developed in animals then injected into the body.

E. A person who harbors a disease-producing organism in the body but does not show signs of the illness is a

(1) Toxoid.
(2) Anaerobe.
(3) Carrier.

F. One disease caused by a virus is

(1) Common cold.
(2) Typhoid fever.
(3) Ringworm.

G. The nurse should know the portals of entry and exit of the common disease-producing organisms because

(1) It will better enable her to pass state board examinations.
(2) It will enable her to aid in the prevention and control of disease.
(3) It will enable her to treat disease in an emergency situation.

H. The body is not protected against disease by

(1) The skin.
(2) Body temperature.
(3) Insulin.

I. The Schick test is given to

(1) Determine the susceptibility to diphtheria.
(2) Diagnose diphtheria.
(3) Treat diphtheria.

J. When disease-producing organisms enter and multiply in the body, the injurious result is

(1) The multiplication of white corpuscles.
(2) The formation of antibodies.
(3) The destruction of tissue.

Aseptic Techniques

DESTROYING DISEASE-PRODUCING MICROORGANISMS

ISOLATION TECHNIQUE

HANDLING STERILE SUPPLIES

REFERENCES

Culver, V.: Modern Bedside Nursing, Chapters 27 and 54.
Hoffman, C. P., Lipkin, G. B., and Thompson, E. M.: Simplified Nursing, pp. 271-282.
Rapier, D. K., et al.: Practical Nursing, pp. 135-142.
Rasmussen, S.: Foundations of Practical and Vocational Nursing, Chapter 17.
Thompson, E. M., and Murphy, C.: Textbook of Basic Nursing, pp. 324-332.

---

1. Complete.

   A. The community water supply is purified by the mechanical means of ________ ________________________________.

   B. The ________________ rays in direct sunlight kill bacteria.

   C. Boiling for __________ minutes makes contaminated articles safe for use.

   D. The only safe method for killing spore-forming organisms is to ____________ __________________ for ________________ minutes.

   E. Cold has the effect of __________________________ microorganisms.

   F. An important point to be remembered when sterilizing articles by boiling is to have the articles completely ____________________ with ____________________ which should be kept ____________________ constantly for the required time.

2. Match each term with the correct definition.

Term		Definition
a. Disinfection	_____	1. Free from all bacteria
b. Asepsis	_____	2. A substance which checks the growth of bacteria
c. Sterile	_____	3. A method which kills disease-producing bacteria
d. Antiseptic	_____	4. A liquid containing a dissolved substance
e. Solution	_____	5. Carrying out procedures to destroy disease-producing organisms

3. Describe the ways in which the following articles can be sterilized:

A. Gauze dressings

B. Bandage scissors

C. Rubber gloves

D. Petrolatum gauze

4. Each of the following statements concerns isolation technique. Correct each statement that is false by crossing out the incorrect word or words and writing the correct word or words in the space above.

A. Medical asepsis means the destruction of pathogenic organisms.

B. The prime purpose of isolation technique is to assist in preventing the spread of communicable disease.

C. A gown should be worn when touching anything that will come in contact with the patient.

D. When entering the isolation unit, put on the gown before the mask.

E. When hanging the gown inside of the isolation unit, hang the contaminated side of the gown on the inside.

F. A mask which is worn properly should cover the nose, mouth and chin.

G. Before putting on a gown, the nurse should push her wrist watch as far up her arm as possible.

H. After wearing a gown in the isolation unit, the entire outside of the gown and the inside of the cuff and neckband are considered contaminated.

I. If there are no hand-washing facilities inside the unit, they should be set up as close to the door as possible.

J. When removing the gown, untie the strings at the neck first.

5. True or False. The following statements refer to handling sterile supplies. Circle T if the statement is true; F if the statement is false.

T F 1. To open a sterile jar, remove the lid and place the lid bottomside down on a flat surface.
T F 2. Alcohol 70 per cent is a sterilizing agent.
T F 3. When using sterile sponge forceps to lift sterile gauze from a can, the entire forceps must remain sterile during the procedure.
T F 4. When handling sterile supplies, never touch sterile articles with unsterile articles.
T F 5. When preparing a dressing cart for use, the dressing forceps should be totally immersed in a sterilizing solution.
T F 6. Supplies are arranged on a dressing cart so that they can be taken from one patient to another without a break in aseptic technique.
T F 7. If sterile supplies become wet, they are contaminated.
T F 8. If one is in doubt as to whether an article is sterile or not, it is safe to use the article providing it looks clean.
T F 9. One may use the fingers to remove alcohol sponges from their container because alcohol is a self-sterilizing solution.
T F 10. A sterile field may be created by covering an area with a sterile towel.
T F 11. Rubber goods may be sterilized by boiling for five minutes.
T F 12. After using a sponge forceps to remove soiled dressings from a wound, it should be dipped in a disinfectant solution before re-using it to apply sterile dressing to the wound.
T F 13. If soiled dressing sticks to a wound, moisten it with tap water until it loosens.
T F 14. When unwrapping a sterile tray, do not touch the inside of the wrap.
T F 15. The nurse should always wash her hands before and after changing dressings.

6. Name five procedures which are done using a sterile technique.

7. Identify and give the purpose of each article shown in Figure 39.

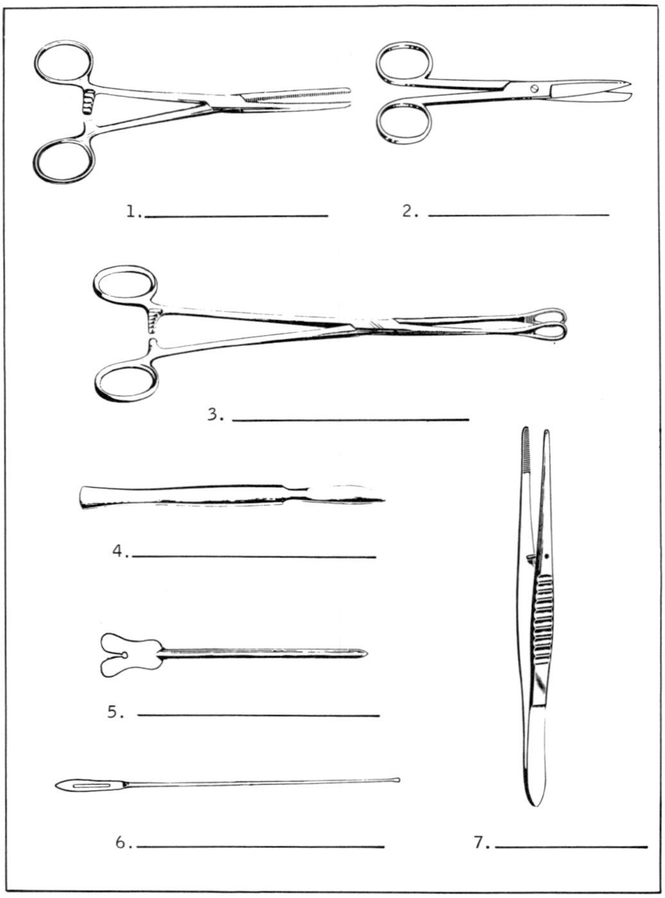

Fig. 39. Surgical instruments. (Dittmar and Penn Corporation, Philadelphia.)

Chapter 30

ADMINISTRATION OF MEDICATIONS

SIMPLE ARITHMETIC
ABBREVIATIONS
SYSTEMS OF WEIGHTS AND MEASURES
METHODS AND RULES OF ADMINISTRATION
TYPES AND ACTIONS OF MEDICATIONS

SIMPLE ARITHMETIC

1. Solve each of the problems.

A. Add:

1786	80	679	8
431	126	11023	189
364	32	6447	47
202	16		35
6			99

B. Subtract:

76	825	365	1728
-43	-178	-96	-976

C. Multiply:

75	36	178	476
x 4	x 17	x 25	x 309

D. Divide:

$4\overline{)128}$ $17\overline{)340}$ $27\overline{)675}$ $86\overline{)1290}$

2. Fractions.

A. A fraction is part of a whole.

B. One-half of a part written as a fraction would be $\frac{1}{2}$.

C. The number above the line is called the numerator.

D. The number below the line is called the denominator.

Example: $\frac{1}{2}$ 1 numerator / 2 denominator

E. Underline the fraction which is the largest part of a whole.

(1) $\frac{3}{4}$ $\frac{2}{4}$ $\frac{1}{5}$ $\frac{7}{8}$

(2) $\frac{5}{6}$ $\frac{4}{7}$ $\frac{3}{10}$ $\frac{1}{5}$

3. Reducing Fractions.

A. To reduce a fraction to the lowest terms, pick any number that will divide into both the numerator and denominator.

Example: $\frac{6}{18}$ divided by $\frac{6}{6}$ equals $\frac{1}{3}$

B. Reduce to the lowest terms:

$\frac{20}{100} =$ $\frac{50}{100} =$ $\frac{75}{100} =$ $\frac{25}{75} =$ $\frac{2}{30} =$

4. Improper fractions and mixed numbers.

A. A proper fraction is a fraction which is less than a whole number.

B. An improper fraction is a fraction in which the numerator is equal to, or larger than, the denominator.

Example: $\frac{7}{5}$ is an improper fraction.

C. A mixed number is a whole number and a fraction.

Example: $7\frac{1}{5}$ is a mixed number.

5. Changing a mixed number to an improper fraction.

A. Multiply the whole number by the denominator of the fraction.

B. Add this to the numerator of the fraction.

C. Place the total over the denominator

Example: $7\frac{1}{5}$ 7 times 5 equals 35 plus 1 equals 36.

The result is $\frac{36}{5}$

D. Change to improper fractions:

$8\frac{3}{4} =$ $6\frac{2}{3} =$ $5\frac{3}{5} =$ $12\frac{1}{2} =$

6. Multiplying whole numbers and fractions.

A. Multiply the whole number by the numerator and place the answer over the denominator.

B. Change the improper fraction to a mixed number by dividing the denominator into the numerator.

Example: $\frac{3}{4}$ of 6 or $\frac{3}{4} \times 6$

$$\frac{3}{4} \times 6 = \frac{18}{4} \qquad 4\overline{)18}\ \text{(quotient 4; } 18 - 16 = 2\text{)} \qquad = 4\frac{2}{4} = 4\frac{1}{2}$$

C. Solve these problems:

$7 \times \frac{3}{4} =$ $\qquad$ $5 \times \frac{2}{3} =$

$12 \times \frac{1}{2} =$ $\qquad$ $25 \times \frac{3}{4} =$

7. Multiplying fractions.

A. Multiply the numerators.

B. Multiply the denominators.

C. Reduce the fraction to its lowest terms.

Example: $\frac{1}{2} \times \frac{2}{3} = \frac{2}{6} = \frac{1}{3}$

D. Solve the following:

$\frac{1}{3} \times \frac{2}{3} =$ $\qquad$ $\frac{1}{6} \times \frac{2}{5} =$

$\frac{7}{8} \times \frac{1}{2} =$ $\qquad$ $\frac{3}{5} \times \frac{1}{4} =$

8. Dividing fractions.

A. Invert the divisor (number by which you divide).

B. Multiply the fraction.

Example: $\frac{3}{4} \div \frac{1}{2}$ $\qquad$ $\frac{3}{4} \times \frac{2}{1} = \frac{6}{4} = 1\frac{1}{2}$

C. Solve the following:

$\frac{3}{4} \div \frac{1}{4} =$ $\qquad$ $\frac{2}{3} \div \frac{1}{2} =$

$\frac{7}{8} \div \frac{1}{6} =$ $\frac{4}{5} \div \frac{2}{3} =$

9. Dividing a mixed number by a fraction.

   A. Change the mixed number to an improper fraction.

   B. Proceed as in dividing fractions.

   C. Solve these:

   $4\frac{1}{2} \div \frac{1}{3} =$

   $2\frac{1}{3} \div \frac{1}{6} =$

10. Dividing a whole number and a fraction.

    A. Place the whole number as the numerator over a denominator of one.

    B. Proceed as in dividing fractions.

    Example: $\frac{1}{2} \div 4$ $\frac{1}{2} \div \frac{4}{1}$ $\frac{1}{2} \times \frac{1}{4} = \frac{1}{8}$

    C. Solve:

    $\frac{1}{3} \div 6 =$

    $6 \div \frac{2}{3} =$

11. Decimals.

    A. Fractions which are part of ten, one hundred, one thousand, etc., may be written as decimals.

    Example: $\frac{1}{10} = .1$

    $\frac{1}{100} = .01$

    $\frac{1}{1000} = .001$

    $6\frac{1}{10} = 6.1$

    $25\frac{25}{100} = 25.25$

B. Change the decimals to fractions:

2.5 =	125.125 =
7.5 =	33.003 =
100.25 =	330.03 =
6.002 =	75.05

C. Underline the number which is the largest.

A. .1, .01, .001

B. .1, .3, .03

C. .250, 2.50, 25.0

D. 12.5, 6.2, 1.25

12. Multiplication of decimals.

A. Count the total number of decimals in both numbers and point off that number in the answer.

Example:	8.25	Two decimal places plus
	x .2	One decimal place equals
	1.650	Three decimal places

B. Solve these:

16.50	1360	14.35	.36
x .20	x .5	x 1.25	x 4.0

13. Division of decimals.

A. Move the decimal to the right of the divisor.

B. Move the decimal the same number of places to the right in the number being divided.

C. Place a decimal directly above that decimal for the answer.

Example: 2.5 ⟌ 7.500

25. ⟌ 7.500

25 ⟌ 75.00

3.00
25 ⟌ 75.00

D. Solve:

$.4\overline{).248}$ $.7\overline{)29.4}$ $.25\overline{)77.50}$

$1.25\overline{).7750}$

14. Roman numerals.

A. Examples:

I = 1	VII = 7	C = 100
II = 2	VIII = 8	D = 500
III = 3	IX = 9	M = 1000
IV = 4	X = 10	
V = 5	XX = 20	
VI = 6	L = 50	

B. Write these numbers in Roman numerals:

17 =	40 =	22 =
19 =	1500 =	75 =
25 =	33 =	15 =

ABBREVIATIONS

REFERENCES

Culver, V.: Modern Bedside Nursing, Appendix I.
Hoffman, C. P., Lipkin, G. B., and Thompson, E. M.: Simplified Nursing, pp. 633-634.
Rapier, D. K., et al.: Practical Nursing, Appendix p. 626.
Rasmussen, S.: Foundations of Practical and Vocational Nursing, pp. 122-123.
Thompson, E. M., and Murphy, C.: Textbook of Basic Nursing, p. 339.

---

1. Rewrite each statement and substitute the correct words for the abbreviations.

   A. Give one tablet p.o. q.4h. for two days then b.i.d.

   B. Give ʒ $\overline{\dot{s}s}$ q.3h. p.r.n. for cough.

   C. Out of bed ad lib.

   D. Give 1 cc. I.M. stat. and repeat h.s. S.O.S.

   E. Give essence of peppermint ʒ 1 c̄ warm water ʒ $\overline{\dot{i}v}$ a.c.

   F. Give S.S. enema p.r.n.

   G. Hot moist saline compresses to the right arm q.i.d.

   H. Weigh q.d. a.c. in A.M.

   I. Give qtts. ī in right eye t.i.d.

   J. Give 20 Gms.^{H} stat.

2. Practice writing the abbreviation for ounce, dram and minim.

Ounce:

Dram:

Minim:

3. In the following statements cross out the words and write the abbreviations above where possible.

A. Give 1 tablet at bedtime.

B. Give aspirin grains five for headache every 4 hours as necessary.

C. Give 5% glucose in water and 5% glucose in saline 1 liter of each every day for two days.

D. Check the blood pressure and pulse every 15 minutes for 4 hours, then every 30 minutes for 12 hours, then every 12 hours for 48 hours.

E. Give 3 cubic centimeters intramuscularly.

SYSTEMS OF WEIGHTS AND MEASURES

When the doctor prescribes any medication for a patient, he always tells you the amount to give. Just as cooking has a system of measurement—i.e., cups, teaspoons, tablespoons—so do medications have special measurements. There are two systems of measurement for medications: the metric system and the apothecaries' system. As you know, drugs can be given in liquid form and solid form. The liquids are measured by pouring a certain amount. The solids are measured by weighing them. There are certain terms or types of measurement for both liquids and solids in both the metric and apothecaries' systems.

METRIC SYSTEM

In the metric system the measurement for liquids is the liter (L.). A liter is the size of a quart. Smaller portions of liquids or solutions are measured by the milliliter (ml.) or by the cubic centimeter (cc.), each of which equals one one-thousandth of a liter. There are 1000 milliliters or 1000 cubic centimeters in 1 liter.

Solve these:

0.5 L. = _____ cc.

0.25 L. = _____ cc.

0.075 L. = _____ ml.

2 L. = _____ cc.

2.5 L. = _____ cc.

Have you noticed that to change liters to cubic centimeters or milliliters, you multiply by 1000?

In the metric system the measurement for solids (weights) is the gram (Gm.). Smaller portions are measured by the milligram (mg.) which equals one one-thousandth of a gram. There are 1000 milligrams in 1 gram.

Solve these:

0.025 Gm. = _____ mg.

0.1 Gm. = _____ mg.

0.064 Gm. = _____ mg.

75 mg. = _____ Gm.

150 mg. = _____ Gm.

Note that in the metric system parts of a whole are always written as decimals rather than as fractions.

THE APOTHECARIES' SYSTEM

In the apothecaries' system the measurement for liquids is a quart (qt.). The quart is broken into pints (pt.), fluid ounces (f℥), fluid drams (f℥), and minims (♏). A minim is about the size of a drop, and a fluid dram is about the size of a teaspoonful.

60 minims = 1 fluid dram

8 fluid drams = 1 fluid ounce

16 fluid ounces = 1 pint

2 pints = 1 quart

Solve these:

1 fluid ounce = _____ fluid drams

1 quart = _____ fluid ounces

1/2 fluid dram = _____ minims

1/2 fluid ounce = _____ fluid dram

Solids or weights are measured in the apothecaries' system by pounds (lb.), ounces (oz.) and grains (gr.). In prescribing solid medications, amounts as large as a pound or an ounce are not used. A grain is used frequently. The weight of one grain is based on the average weight of a grain of wheat.

USING BOTH THE METRIC AND APOTHECARIES' SYSTEMS

Amounts of drugs are prepared and prescribed using both the metric and apothecaries' systems. For example, a tablet may contain a certain number of grams (metric) of aspirin. The same is true in using liquid drugs. The doctor may order, for example, cough medicine to be given in a certain number of fluid drams (apothecaries') or a certain number of cubic centimeters (metric).

The label on a bottle of tablets may state that each tablet contains so many grains of a drug, but when the doctor writes an order, he may ask you to give so many grams of the drug. Since a grain and a gram are not the same size, you would have to figure out the dosage to give.

Here are the equivalents of the metric and apothecaries' systems. The liquid household system is shown for comparison.

Weight Measures

Metric	Apothecaries'
60 milligrams or 0.06 gram	1 grain
1 gram	15 grains
4 grams	1 dram
30 grams	1 ounce

Liquid Measures

Metric	Apothecaries'	
1 cubic centimeter	15 minims	15 drops
4 cubic centimeters	1 fluid dram	1 teaspoon
30 cubic centimeters	1 fluid ounce	8 teaspoons or 2 tablespoons
500 cubic centimeters	1 pint	2 cups
1000 cubic centimeters	1 quart	4 cups

Learn the metric, apothecaries' and household systems of weights and measures and solve these problems:

1. 1 dram = __________ cubic centimeters
2. 1 gram = __________ grains.
3. 1 cubic centimeter = __________ minims.
4. 1 teaspoon = __________ drams.
5. 1 quart = __________ cubic centimeters.
6. 1 fluid ounce = __________ cubic centimeters.
7. 1 fluid ounce = __________ fluid drams.
8. 2 cups = __________ pints.
9. 1/2 cubic centimeter = __________ minims.
10. 2 grams = __________ grains.
11. 1/2 gram = __________ grains.
12. 8 cubic centimeters = __________ fluid drams.
13. 180 cubic centimeters = __________ fluid ounces.
14. 1000 cubic centimeters = __________ fluid ounces.
15. 4 cups = __________ cubic centimeters.
16. 75 grains = __________ grams.
17. $\overline{ss}$ grams = __________ grains.
18. 1/3 cubic centimeter = __________ minims.
19. 1 fluid dram = __________ minims.
20. 1 pint = __________ quarts.

21. Aspirin gr. X is ordered: Each tablet equals gr. V. Give ____________ tablets.

22. Penicillin 600,000 units is ordered. Each cc. equals 300,000 units.

Give ____________ cc.

23. Gantrisin gr. $\overline{\dot{v}\dot{i}\dot{i}ss}$ is ordered. Each tablet equals Gm. $\overline{\dot{i}}$. Give ________ tablets.

24. Streptomycin Gm. $\overline{\dot{s}s}$ is ordered. 1 cc. equals Gm. 1. Give ______________ cc.

25. Ferrous sulfate gr. X is ordered. Each tablet equals gr. V. Give ______________ tablets.

26. Aspirin 0.6 Gm. is ordered. Each tablet contains gr. $\overline{\dot{v}}$. Give ________ tablets.

27. Phenobarbital 0.03 Gm. is ordered. Each tablet contains 1/4 gr. Give __________ tablet.

28. Phenobarbital 30 mg. is ordered. Each tablet contains 1/4 gr. Give ___________ tablet.

29. Codeine sulfate 0.015 Gm. is ordered. Each tablet contains 1/4 gr. Give_______ tablet.

30. 0.6 Gm. is ordered. Each tablet contains 20 gr. Give ________ tablet.

METHODS AND RULES OF ADMINISTRATION

REFERENCES

Culver, V.: Modern Bedside Nursing, Chapter 30.
Hoffman, C. P., Lipkin, G. B., and Thompson, E. M.: Simplified Nursing, Chapter 24.
Rapier, D. K., et al.: Practical Nursing, Chapters 33 and 34.
Rasmussen, S.: Foundations of Practical and Vocational Nursing, Chapter 18.
Thompson, E. M., and Murphy, C.: Textbook of Basic Nursing, pp. 334-352.

JOURNALS

Morris, William E.: Parenteral fluid therapy. J. Practical Nursing, 16:32, Sept. 1966.
Spring, Maxwell: Injections – intramuscular and subcutaneous. Bedside Nurse, 1:17, July-Aug. 1968.

1. List the reasons why each route of administration is used to give drugs:

   A. Oral

   B. Injection

   C. Topical

   D. Inhalation

2. Figure 40 shows a medicine cabinet with bottles of drugs and a medicine tray with name cards. Assume that you have been assigned to pouring these medications. On the line below each medicine card, write the number of the bottle of medication you would use from the medicine cabinet. Next to the number, write the number of tablets or cubic centimeters you would give the patient.

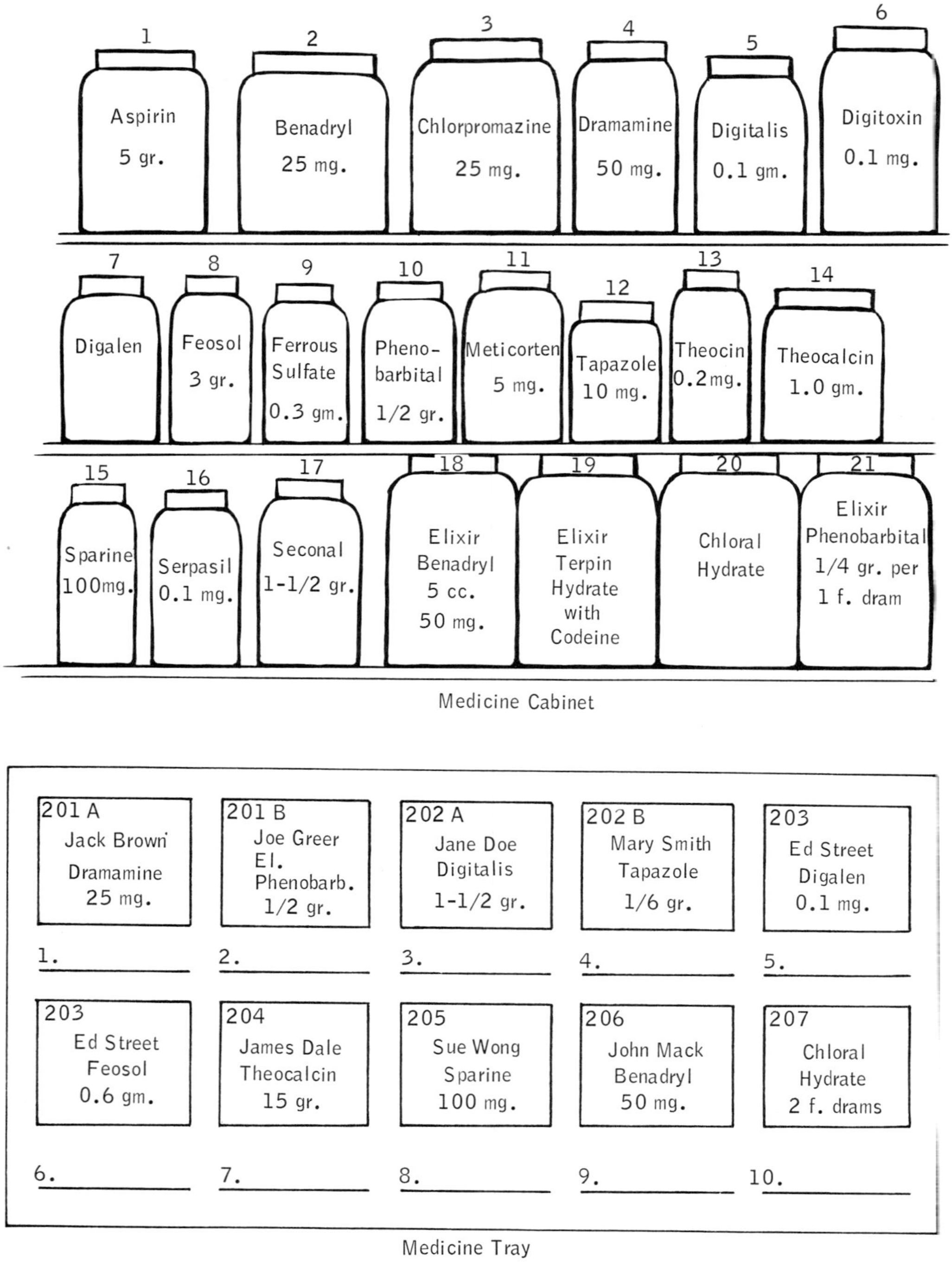

Fig. 40. Medicine Tray.

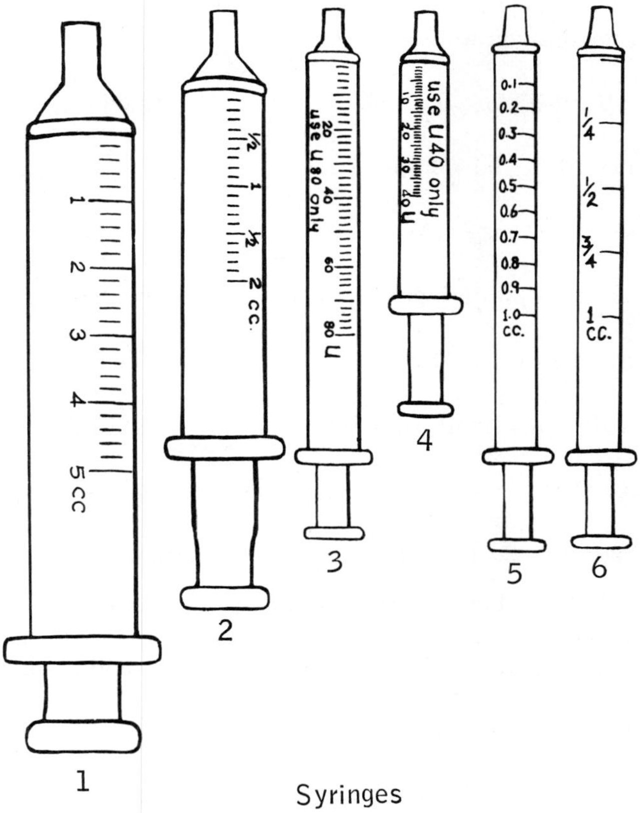

Syringes

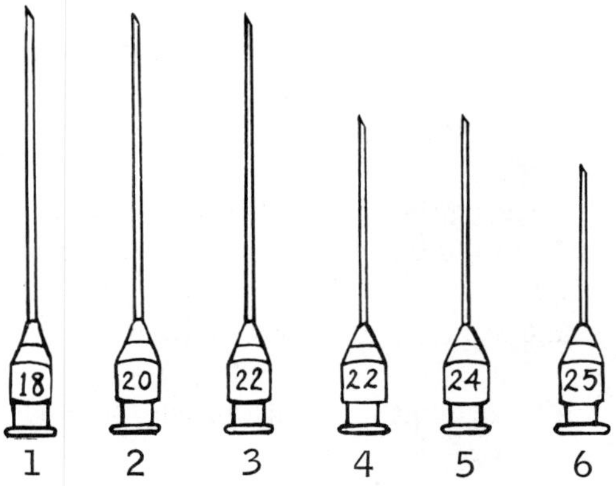

Needles

Fig. 41. Needles.

3. You are assigned to give several injections. In Figure 41 select the number of the syringe and needle you would use.

A. Give penicillin 300,000 U. I.M.	Needle ________
On hand penicillin 100,000 per cc.	Syringe ________
B. Give Demerol 100 mg. I.M.	Needle ________
On hand Demerol 50 mg. per cc.	Syringe ________
C. Give regular insulin U. 30.	Needle ________
On hand regular insulin 40 U. per cc.	Syringe ________

4. Multiple choice. Circle the number preceding the answer.

A. When giving a needle injection, the following should be sterile:

(1) Plunger, outside of barrel and needle.
(2) Needle hub, plunger and outside of barrel.
(3) Needle cannula, inside of barrel, barrel tip and plunger.

B. Several "don'ts" in giving medications are

a. Don't give a medication from an unlabeled container.	1. a, b, c
b. Never give a medication unless you know the manufacturer's name.	2. b, d, e
c. Don't put liquids back in the bottle after being poured.	3. All but b
d. Never give a medication someone else has prepared.	4. All
e. Never leave the medicine within the reach of the patient.	5. c, d, e

C. Some advantages of giving medications hypodermically are

a. The patient can be forced to take a medication he may otherwise refuse.	1. all but d
b. To obtain a more rapid action of a drug.	2. b, d, e
c. To administer a medication that may be destroyed by digestive juices.	3. a, b, d, e
d. In some instances, it is more convenient for the nurse.	4. b, c, e
e. It enables the treatment of a patient who is unable to take oral medications.	5. All

D. The dangers to the patient in giving a needle injection are

a. Infection.	1. a, c, d
b. Damage to the tissues.	2. b, c, d
c. Striking a nerve	3. None
d. Injecting the fluid into a blood vessel.	4. All

E. To withdraw medication from an ampule

a. Before filing, shake all the solution from the narrow end of the ampule	1. a, c, d
b. Inject air into the ampule before withdrawing the solution.	2. a, c, d
c. Protect fingers with gauze when breaking the ampule.	3. All
d. Avoid touching the needle to the outside of the ampule.	4. c

F. When giving an intramuscular injection

a. Hold the syringe at a 30 degree angle to the skin.	1. a, c, e
b. Use a short needle.	2. c, d, e
c. The best site for the injection is in the upper quadrant of the buttocks.	3. All but a
d. Hold the syringe perpendicular to the skin.	4. c
e. Always use a 10 cc. syringe.	5. c, d

G. When giving cough medicine

(1) Give through a drinking tube to prevent irritation to the mucous membranes.
(2) Give with ice to lessen the unpleasant taste.
(3) Give undiluted to get the maximum effect.

H. Insulin is administered

a. Subcutaneously.	1. a, b, d
b. With an insulin syringe.	2. All but e
c. With a needle less than an inch long.	3. b, c, d
d. In dosages of Units.	4. All but c
e. At a different site each time.	5. All

I. If a patient refuses to take a medication,

a. Tell him his attitude is quite childish.	1. a, c, e
b. Inform him that if he wishes to be uncooperative you have the right to refuse to care for him.	2. d
c. Report the incident to the doctor or charge nurse.	3. e
d. Do or say nothing if it happens only once.	4. c
e. Chart the refusal.	5. c, e

J. The list of official drugs that is published is the

(1) New and Nonofficial Drugs.
(2) The United States Pharmacopeia.
(3) Harrison Narcotic Law.

TYPES AND ACTIONS OF MEDICATIONS

REFERENCES

Culver, V.: Modern Bedside Nursing, Chapter 31.
Hoffman, C. P., Lipkin, G. B., and Thompson, E. M.: Simplified Nursing, Appendix p. 595.
Rapier, D. K., et al.: Practical Nursing, Chapter 35.
Rasmussen, S.: Foundations of Practical and Vocational Nursing, Appendix 2, p. 691.
Thompson, E. M., and Murphy, C.: Textbook of Basic Nursing, pp. 352-386.

1. Match each drug action with the correct definition.

Action		Definition
a. Stimulant	_____	1. Produces bowel movements
b. Depressant	_____	2. Relieves nervous tension
c. Antibiotic	_____	3. Checks the growth of bacteria
d. Cathartic	_____	4. Neutralizes gastrointestinal acids
e. Expectorant	_____	5. Increases the amount of urine secreted
f. Sedative	_____	6. Lessens the function of organs
g. Analgesic	_____	7. Destroys microorganisms
h. Diuretic	_____	8. Increases the activity of organs
i. Antacid	_____	9. Relieves pain
j. Disinfectant	_____	10. Loosens bronchial secretions

2. Match each drug with its correction action.

Drug		Action
a. Barbiturates	_____	1. Cathartic
b. Aspirin	_____	2. Antibiotic
c. Sodium bicarbonate	_____	3. Disinfectant
d. Caffeine	_____	4. Analgesic
e. Cascara	_____	5. Antacid
f. Penicillin	_____	6. Anticoagulant
g. Ether	_____	7. Stimulant
h. Zephiran chloride	_____	8. Expectorant
i. Dicumarol	_____	9. Sedative
j. Elixir terpin hydrate	_____	10. Anesthetic

3. Match each drug with the condition for which it is commonly used.

Drug		Condition
a. Serpasil	______	1. Heart failure
b. Digitalis	______	2. Gastric ulcer
c. Heparin	______	3. Hypertension
d. Menadione	______	4. Constipation
e. Novobiocin	______	5. Staphylococci infection
f. PAS	______	6. Blood clot
g. Amphojel	______	7. Edema
h. Liquid petrolatum	______	8. Urinary tract infection
i. Sulfonamides	______	9. Tuberculosis
j. Diamox	______	10. Deficiency in blood clotting

PART VI

THE MEDICAL AND SURGICAL PATIENT

Chapter 31

INTRODUCTION TO ILLNESS CONDITIONS

DEFINITIONS
TYPES, CAUSES AND BODY REACTIONS TO DISEASE

REFERENCES

Culver, V.: Modern Bedside Nursing, Chapter 40.
Hoffman, C. P., Lipkin, G. P., and Thompson, E. M.: Simplified Nursing, Chapter 27.
Johnston, D. F.: Total Patient Care, 2nd ed. St. Louis, The C. V. Mosby Co., 1968, Chapters 1 and 2.
Keane, C. B.: Essentials of Nursing, Chapter 2.
Mason, M. A.: Basic Medical and Surgical Nursing. 2nd ed. New York, The Macmillan Co., 1967, Chapters 1-4.
Rapier, D. K., et al.: Practical Nursing, Chapter 42.
Thompson, E., and Murphy, C.: Textbook of Basic Nursing, Chapter 32.

As an introduction to the study of illness conditions, it is helpful to become acquainted first with some of the basic terminology, or common words, used to describe various conditions. You have already learned that the medical profession has a language of its own and that it is necessary for the nurse to understand the commonly used words. If you learn certain word endings, it will be easy to tell what the word means. For example, the following is a list of common word endings and the definition of each:

-ology - study of

-ectomy - surgical removal of

-itis - inflammation of

-otomy - surgical opening into

-ostomy - the creation of an artificial opening into

These endings, then, are combined with words to make new terms as follows:

laryngology - the study of the larynx

laryngitis - inflammation of the larynx

laryngotomy - the surgical opening of the larynx

laryngectomy - the surgical removal of the larynx

laryngostomy - the formation of an artificial opening into the larynx

Larynx is an easy word to use because it pertains to the anatomic structure, the larynx. Here is a list of terms for other parts of the body you will be using frequently:

cholecystic - pertaining to the gallbladder

cystic - pertaining to the urinary bladder

dermatic - pertaining to the skin

gastric - pertaining to the stomach

hystero - pertaining to the uterus

nephric - pertaining to the kidney

neuro - pertaining to the nerves

When using these terms to form new words by combining them with the word endings, the letters ic are dropped.

Example:	gastritis	gastrotomy
	gastrectomy	gastrostomy

1. Write the definition of each word

   A. Nephritis

   B. Gynecology

   C. Dermatitis

   D. Cholecystectomy

   E. Tracheotomy

   F. Pharmacology

2. Join the proper terms and word endings to make these words

   A. A study of the skin

   B. Inflammation of the appendix

   C. Inflammation of the urinary bladder

   D. The surgical removal of the kidney

   E. Inflammation of the colon

F. An artificial opening into the colon

G. An incision into the ileum

H. Inflammation of the bronchial tube

I. The surgical removal of the uterus

J. The study of the nerves

3. Match each term with the correct definition.

Term		Definition
a. Illness	_____	1. Caused by injury
b. Congenital	_____	2. Rapid in onset
c. Infectious	_____	3. Swelling
d. Traumatic	_____	4. Limited to one area
e. Local	_____	5. Treatment
f. Acute	_____	6. Present at birth
g. Therapy	_____	7. A condition which prohibits a particular treatment
h. Edema		
i. Predisposing	_____	8. Caused by bacteria
j. Contraindicate	_____	9. A disturbance of the normal functions of the body
	_____	10. Showing a tendency toward a certain illness

4. Rewrite each sentence using the proper medical terminology whenever possible.

A. She has a cardiac condition which appeared suddenly and caused severe pain in the heart area.

B. This blindness was not due to injury, but was present at birth.

C. Race or age may be a factor in a person's having a tendency toward certain illnesses.

5. What observation should the nurse make regarding a patient's pain?

6. Multiple Choice. Circle the number preceding the correct answer. Each question has only one correct answer.

A. An increase in the white blood cell count is called

(1) Erythrocytosis..
(2) Leukocytosis.
(3) Monocytosis.

B. Symptoms which usually accompany an elevated temperature are

(1) Increased pulse and respiration rate.
(2) Elevated blood pressure and pulse rate.
(3) Tachycardia and dyspnea.

C. The redness which occurs in a local inflammation is caused by

(1) The pressure on nerve endings.
(2) An accumulation of fluid in the tissues.
(3) An increase in circulation.

D. A clear watery discharge from tissue is called

(1) Serous exudate.
(2) Bloody exudate.
(3) Suppuration.

E. The death of a tissue is called

(1) Slough.
(2) Necrosis.
(3) Adhesion.

F. Difficult respirations are called

(1) Dyspnea.
(2) Apnea.
(3) Orthopnea.

G. Symptoms which are felt only by the patient are called

(1) Objective.
(2) Subjective.
(3) Acute.

H. A tumor growth could be classified as

(1) A neoplastic disease.
(2) A deficiency disease.
(3) An allergic disease.

I. The lay term "proud flesh" refers to

(1) The formation of scar tissue.
(2) Adhesions.
(3) A laceration.

J. A bluish discoloration of the skin, lips or nails is called

(1) Anemia.
(2) Emesis.
(3) Cyanosis.

Chapter 32

CARING FOR THE CANCER PATIENT

REFERENCES

Culver, V.: Modern Bedside Nursing, Chapter 42.
Hoffman, C. P., Lipkin, G. P., and Thompson, E. M.: Simplified Nursing, Chapter 29.
Johnston, D. F.: Total Patient Care, Chapter 6.
Keane, C. B.: Essentials of Nursing, Chapter 9.
Mason, M. A.: Basic Medical and Surgical Nursing, Chapter 7.
Rapier, D. K., et al.: Practical Nursing, pp. 402-404.
Thompson, E., and Murphy, C.: Textbook of Basic Nursing, Chapter 37.

JOURNALS

Bouchard, Rosemary: The LPN in uterine cancer nursing. J. Practical Nursing, 16:33, April 1966.
Lung cancer: implications for nursing care. J. Practical Nursing, 18:20, Aug. 1968.

A tumor is an independent growth of new tissue. A tumor may be either benign or malignant. A benign tumor is one which does not destroy body tissue. An example of a benign tumor is a wart. A malignant tumor is a lawless growth of cells which destroys body tissue. Cancer is a malignant tumor. There are several kinds of cancers.

1. True or False: Circle T if the statement is true; F if the statement is false.

T F 1. The belief that cancer is contagious has recently been scientifically proven to be true.
T F 2. The majority of tumors are malignant.
T F 3. Cancer is the second leading cause of death in the United States.
T F 4. There are several patent medicines on the market that aid in checking the growth of a malignancy.
T F 5. The diet in cancer should be high in protein.
T F 6. Hodgkin's disease is a malignancy of lymphatic tissue.
T F 7. The diagnosis of cancer is made by a microscopic examination of a frozen section of tissue.
T F 8. Terminal cancer is cancer which has been diagnosed early and cured.
T F 9. A gastrostomy is an artificial anus.
T F 10. Most patients who have cancer have many absurd fears.

2. Multiple Choice. Circle the number preceding the correct answer to each statement.

A. A person over thirty-five years of age should have a physical examination for cancer detection

(1) Once every six months.
(2) Once yearly.
(3) Once every two years.

B. A malignancy of the blood is called

(1) Anemia.
(2) Leukemia.
(3) Hodgkin's disease.

C. In the nursing care of the patient receiving x-ray therapy, the skin over the area being treated

(1) Should be rubbed frequently with alcohol.
(2) Should be bathed frequently.
(3) Should not be bathed with soap and water.

D. The skin over the area receiving x-ray therapy may become

(1) Reddened, tender and itchy.
(2) Cold and clammy.
(3) Show no change.

E. The practical nurse can best help the attitudes of the cancer patient by

(1) Maintaining a sympathetic attitude.
(2) Exercising efficiency and skill when performing her duties.
(3) Maintaining a cheerful, matter-of-fact attitude.

F. A diet high in proteins would include large portions of foods such as

(1) Yellow fruits and vegetables.
(2) Milk, meat and eggs.
(3) Green leafy vegetables.

G. Proteins are necessary in the body to

(1) Build and repair tissue.
(2) Maintain the acid-base balance.
(3) Stimulate the secretion of hormones.

H. For the patient who has a colostomy, it is often necessary to regulate the diet to prevent

(1) Nausea.
(2) Diarrhea.
(3) Dyspepsia.

I. The best contribution the practical nurse can make toward the rehabilitation of the patient with a colostomy is

(1) Helping the patient to understand that a colostomy is not a disabling condition.
(2) Assisting the patient in doing the colostomy irrigations.
(3) Leaving the patient alone as much as possible so that he can have sufficient time to think about a solution to his problems.

J. A medication given to relieve pain is called an

(1) Antibiotic.
(2) Antacid.
(3) Analgesic.

K. The surgical removal of a breast is called a

(1) Mastectomy.
(2) Gastrectomy.
(3) Mastoidectomy.

L. All persons who have a permanent tracheostomy

(1) Will have to be fed through a tube the rest of their lives.
(2) Are visibly disfigured.
(3) Must learn to talk again.

M. When dressings must be changed frequently, it is best to hold them in place with adhesive strips called

(1) Band aids.
(2) Montgomery tapes.
(3) Ace bandage.

N. The nurse can help in preventing irritation to the skin around a colostomy stoma by

(1) Giving frequent colostomy irrigations.
(2) Forcing fluids.
(3) Keeping the skin clean.

O. A substance used as a deodorizing agent is

(1) Chloral hydrate.
(2) Fluorine.
(3) Chlorophyll.

3. Discussion.

A. While you are bathing Mrs. B., a patient with carcinoma of the cervix, she asks, "Do I have cancer?" How will you reply?

B. Mr. X., a patient with terminal cancer, asks, "Am I going to die?" How will you reply?

C. Miss M. has been admitted to the hospital for diagnostic studies. Her symptoms are occasional rectal bleeding associated with diarrhea. She is quite depressed and states, "My mother had this very same trouble and she died of cancer four years ago. I guess I'm following in her footsteps." How can you help Miss M.?

D. Mrs. E. has had a radical mastectomy. Several days after surgery, she asks your advice concerning a prosthesis. What can you tell her?

E. Your next door neighbor approaches you saying, "I think it is absolutely shameful that doctors don't tell patients they have cancer." What will your reply be?

Chapter 33

THE ELDERLY PATIENT

REFERENCES

Culver, V.: Modern Bedside Nursing, Chapter 50.
Hoffman, C. P., Lipkin, G. P., and Thompson, E. M.: Simplified Nursing, Chapter 26.
Johnston, D. F.: Total Patient Care, Chapter 8.
Keane, C. B.: Essentials of Nursing, Chapter 7.
Rapier, D. K., et al.: Practical Nursing, Chapters 43 and 45.
Stevens, M. K.: Geriatric Nursing for Practical Nurses. Philadelphia, W. B. Saunders Co., 1965.

JOURNALS

Routh, Thomas A.: Anxiety in geriatric nursing. Am. J. Practical Nursing, 2:108, May 1966.
Verwoerdt, Adriaan: Psychological factors in geriatric nursing care. J. Practical Nursing, 17:24, Feb. 1967.

Remember: Old age in itself is not a disease!

1. Explain why each of the following should be part of the nursing care for the elderly patient:

A. Encouraging the patient to do as much for himself as possible

B. Protecting the patient from environmental hazards

C. Providing warmth

D. Providing for originality and variation in the daily menu

E. Providing early morning snacks when permitted

2. Multiple Choice. Circle the number preceding the correct answer to each statement.

A. The branch of medicine concerned with the care of the aged is called

(1) Geriatrics.
(2) Pediatrics.
(3) Orthopedics.

B. The leading cause of death in the United States is

(1) Cancer.
(2) Heart disease.
(3) Accidents.

C. The most important aspect in the nurse-patient relationship when caring for the elderly patient is for the nurse to

(1) Treat the patient the same as she would a child.
(2) Always speak loudly and clearly to the patient because most elderly persons are hard of hearing.
(3) Realize that elderly persons have the same basic needs as persons of all ages.

D. The percentage of persons over the age of sixty-five who have no regular income is

(1) Over 10 per cent.
(2) Over 25 per cent.
(3) Over 50 per cent.

E. The Social Security Administration is a division of the United States Department of

(1) Agriculture.
(2) Health, Education, and Welfare.
(3) Public Health.

F. Elderly persons like best to associate with

(1) Persons their own age.
(2) Younger persons.
(3) No one.

G. Many elderly persons fail to eat their daily requirement of foods containing proteins because

(1) They cannot chew properly.
(2) They dislike these types of foods.
(3) They cannot afford them.

H. The aged patient would most enjoy talking about his

(1) Plans for the future.
(2) Past experiences.
(3) Present-day life.

I. In the nursing care of the chronically ill, good skin care is a must in the prevention of

(1) Aging skin.
(2) Edema.
(3) Decubitus ulcers.

J. The skin of the elderly patient should be rubbed with

(1) Alcohol.
(2) Powder.
(3) Cold cream.

K. The usual sleeping habit of the aged is that of

(1) Going to bed late and rising early.
(2) Going to bed early and rising early.
(3) Going to bed early and rising late.

L. A good rule for the nurse to follow when caring for a patient whose habits are deeply ingrained is to

(1) Make the patient understand in the initial care that you will be the boss.
(2) Explain to the patient that you are at his service and will comply with his wishes.
(3) Help the patient alter only those habits which will harm his well-being.

M. When planning diversional therapy for an aged person, one should first understand his

(1) Mental and physical capacity.
(2) Personal hygiene habits.
(3) Financial status.

N. The nurse must be careful in observing and recording the bowel habits of the bedridden elderly patient because

(1) It is usually a strictly enforced hospital procedure.
(2) Inactivity tends to cause constipation.
(3) Most elderly persons are incontinent of feces.

O. An abnormal mental condition that occurs in the latter years of life is called

(1) Senile dementia.
(2) Schizophrenia.
(3) Multiple sclerosis.

Chapter 34

DISEASES OF THE DIGESTIVE SYSTEM

ANATOMY AND PHYSIOLOGY REVIEW
DIAGNOSTIC EXAMINATIONS
DISEASE CONDITIONS: GASTRITIS, PEPTIC ULCER, GALLBLADDER DISEASES, APPENDICITIS, COLITIS, HERNIA, INTESTINAL OBSTRUCTION, HEMORRHOIDS, LIVER DISEASES
GENERAL NURSING CARE

REFERENCES

Culver, V.: Modern Bedside Nursing, Chapters 11 and 44.
Hoffman, C. P., Lipkin, G. P., and Thompson, E. M.: Simplified Nursing, Chapter 34.
Johnston, D. F.: Total Patient Care, Chapter 13.
Keane, C. B.: Essentials of Nursing, Chapter 14.
Mason, M. A.: Basic Medical and Surgical Nursing, Chapters 14-16.
Rapier, D. K., et al.: Practical Nursing, pp. 408-413.
Thompson, E., and Murphy, C.: Textbook of Basic Nursing, Chapter 38.

ANATOMY AND PHYSIOLOGY REVIEW

1. Label the parts of the digestive system on Figure 42.

   A. Label:

   (1) Esophagus
   (2) Stomach
   (3) Liver
   (4) Pylorus
   (5) Pancreas
   (6) Duodenum
   (7) Ileum
   (8) Jejunum
   (9) Appendix
   (10) Cecum
   (11) Colon
   (12) Rectum

   B. Color:

   (1) Gallbladder - brown
   (2) Common bile duct - red
   (3) Salivary glands - yellow

2. Match each organ of the digestive system with its correct function.

Organ		Function
a. Gallbladder	______	1. Secretes gastric juices
b. Esophagus	______	2. Stores bile
c. Liver	______	3. Mixes food with saliva
d. Stomach	______	4. A food passageway
e. Tongue	______	5. Manufactures bile

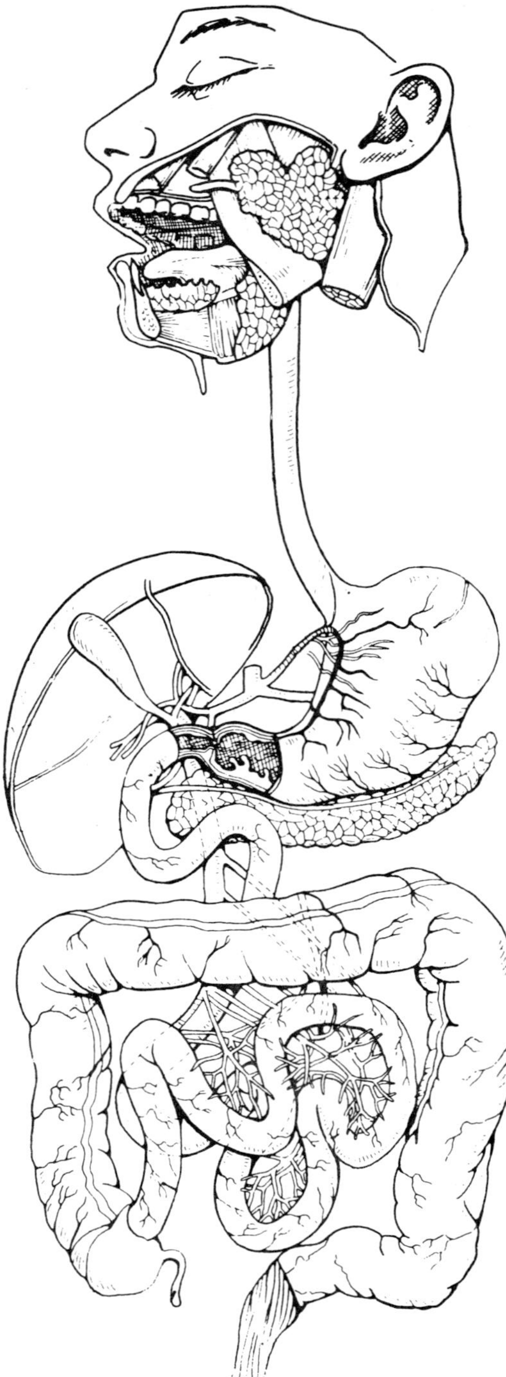

Fig. 42. Digestive system. (Denoyer-Geppert Company, Chicago, Illinois.)

EXAMINATION	DEFINITION	PREPARATION OF PATIENT	RESPONSIBILITIES OF PRACTICAL NURSE
Gastrointestinal series			
Cholecystogram			
Barium enema			
Sigmoidoscopic examination			
Gastric analysis			
Gastroscopic examination			

COMMON DISEASES OF THE DIGESTIVE SYSTEM

1. Gastritis is inflammation of the stomach. The inflammation may be either acute or chronic.

	ACUTE	CHRONIC
Cause		
Symptoms		
Treatment		
Nursing care		

2. Peptic Ulcer. An ulcer is the localized destruction of tissue on a cutaneous or mucous surface. A peptic ulcer is an ulcer which occurs in the portion of the digestive tract that is exposed to the acidic gastric juices. Peptic ulcers occur most commonly in the duodenum and next most frequently in the stomach. Ulcers vary in size, shape and depth; some involve only the mucous membrane, others extend into the muscular lining and still others may perforate through all the linings of the organ.

A. Describe the pain associated with peptic ulcers.

B. What complications may develop if a peptic ulcer perforates?

C. What may the presence of tarry stools signify?

D. Medical treatment of the peptic ulcer consists of rest, diet and antacids.

(1) Why is rest important?

(2) Name two antacid preparations which are frequently used.

(3) Explain the regime used in the Sippy diet.

(4) List the instructions which should be given to the peptic ulcer patient upon discharge from the hospital. Why?

E. When is it necessary to treat the peptic ulcer surgically?

3. Gallbladder Diseases. The gallbladder or bile ducts, or both, may become inflamed. Gallstones may form in the gallbladder and transport to the cystic duct or common bile duct. Gallstones vary in size, shape and number.

A. Define:

(1) Cholecystitis

(2) Cholelithiasis

(3) Cholecystectomy

B. List the symptoms of cholecystitis

C. What causes jaundice in gallbladder disease?

D. Outline a day's menu for a fat free diet.

4. Appendicitis is inflammation of the appendix. The walls of the appendix become inflamed and the organ often fills with pus.

A. Symptoms:

B. Treatment:

C. Complications:

D. Name two measures which are contraindicated for anyone suspected of having the symptoms of appendicitis.

5. Colitis is inflammation of the colon. The most frequent infections of the colon are amebic and bacillary dysentery. Colitis may also be secondary to cancer.

A. Symptoms:

B. Medical Treatment:

C. Surgical Treatment:

6. Hernia, or rupture, is a protrusion of a portion of the contents of a cavity through a weakness in its wall. Hernia may occur in various parts of the body; however, the term usually applies to the varieties which affect the abdominal wall. In this case, a loop of the intestine pushes through a weak spot in the muscular wall of the abdomen.

A. Symptoms:

B. Treatment:

7. Intestinal obstruction is a blocking of the intestinal tract. The intestinal passage may be partially or completely blocked. Intestinal obstruction is really a symptom rather than a disease.

A. What conditions may cause an intestinal obstruction?

B. Symptoms:

C. Treatment:

D. Define:

(1) Enterostomy:

(2) Intestinal resection:

8. Hemorrhoids, or piles, are varicose veins of the lower part of the rectum and anal canal. When they are located at the junction of the rectum and anal canal, they are called internal hemorrhoids; when they are in the region of the anal opening, they are called external hemorrhoids. Very often the patient has both types.

A. Symptoms:

B. Treatment:

9. Liver Diseases. Inflammation of the liver is called hepatitis. Hepatitis frequently occurs epidemically. Another disease, in which liver cells are destroyed and replaced by scar tissue, is called cirrhosis of the liver. Most diseases of the liver are treated medically.

A. How do the symptoms differ in these two conditions?

B. Discuss the diet used in treating liver disease.

C. Define ascites and explain the procedure which is performed to relieve this condition.

GENERAL NURSING CARE

A. Multiple Choice. Circle the number preceding the correct answer to each statement.

Mr. K. was admitted to the hospital for a hemorrhoidectomy. Prior to surgery he was to receive a tap water cleansing enema.

(1) In giving the enema, the nurse will use precautions to prevent rectal discomfort by

(a) Administering only 100 cc. solution.
(b) Using a small, well-lubricated rectal tube.
(c) Allowing the patient to give his own enema.

(2) Following surgery Mr. K. received sitz baths three times daily. The reasons for this procedure could best be explained to the patient by saying

(a) "This will help to relieve pain and aid in healing."
(b) "This will prevent constipation."
(c) "It is given to cleanse the perineum."

(3) The charge nurse asked the student practical nurse to get Mr. K. a clean binder to hold his dressings in place. The type binder used would be

(a) Scultetus binder.
(b) Abdominal binder.
(c) "T" binder.

Mr. S. returned to his room following a partial gastrectomy. He had a Levin tube in place, which was connected to a Wangensteen suction apparatus.

(4) The purpose of the Wangensteen suction is to

(a) Administer food to the body.
(b) Drain fluids from the stomach, thus preventing abdominal distention.
(c) Prevent retention of urine.

(5) The Levin tube was irrigated with sterile water every two hours in order to

(a) Prevent the Levin tube from becoming clogged.
(b) Promote rapid healing of the operative site.
(c) Supply fluids to the body.

(6) For the first 48 hours postoperatively Mr. S. was allowed nothing by mouth. During this time, the patient complained of "dryness in the mouth." In order to relieve this discomfort, the practical nurse would

(a) Give him a few sips of water.
(b) Explain to him that he would have to learn to tolerate this since nothing could be done to offer relief.
(c) Swab the mouth with a mixture of glycerin and lemon juice.
(d) Do none of these.

(7) The patient has an order for morphine sulfate gr. 1/6 Ⓗ when needed. This drug is given for its action as an

(a) Analgesic.
(b) Antibiotic.
(c) Antacid.

(8) The nurse can do the following to aid in the comfort of the patient:

(a) Avoid noise and confusion.
(b) Insure proper ventilation of the room.
(c) Keep the patient's position comfortable.
(d) None of these.
(e) All of these.

(9) When inserting a flatus tube, the following items would not be needed:

(a) Small rectal tube and lubricant.
(b) Urinal and cover.
(c) Irrigating can and rubber tubing.

(10) In administering a gastrostomy feeding, the following is not done:

(a) Have the feeding at body temperature.
(b) Administer the feeding rapidly.
(c) Administer a small amount of tap water after giving the feeding.

B. Discussion. Explain how the practical nurse can contribute to the nursing care of diseases of the digestive system in the following areas:

1. Health teaching

2. Diversional therapy

3. Observation of symptoms

C. Medication Review.

1. Match each drug with its action.

Action		Drug
a. Antacid	_____	1. Ipecac
b. Emetic	_____	2. Thorazine
c. Antiemetic	_____	3. Cascara
d. Cathartic	_____	4. Amphojel
e. Antispasmodic	_____	5. Kaopectate
f. Antidiarrheic	_____	6. Dramamine
	_____	7. Gelusil
	_____	8. Banthine
	_____	9. Magnesium sulfate
	_____	10. Tincture of belladonna

2. List several points that are essential in the method of giving dilute hydrochloric acid.

Chapter 35

ORTHOPEDIC NURSING

ANATOMY AND PHYSIOLOGY REVIEW
DISEASE CONDITIONS: FRACTURES, OSTEOMYELITIS, RICKETS, BURSITIS, DISLOCATIONS, MUSCULAR DYSTROPHY, SPRAINS, SARCOMA, ARTHRITIS
GENERAL NURSING CARE

REFERENCES

Culver, V.: Modern Bedside Nursing, Chapters 7, 8 and 43.
Hoffman, C. P., Lipkin, G. P., and Thompson, C. M.: Simplified Nursing, Chapter 31.
Johnston, D. F.: Total Patient Care, Chapter 20.
Keane, C. B.: Essentials of Nursing, Chapter 11.
Mason, M. A.: Basic Medical and Surgical Nursing, Chapter 17.
Rapier, D. K., et al.: Practical Nursing, pp. 398-399 and 422-424.
Thompson, E., and Murphy, C.: Textbook of Basic Nursing, Chapter 35.

JOURNALS

Clark, William S.: Arthritis: a challenge to excellence in nursing care. J. Practical Nursing, 18:23, May 1968.
Helfand, Arthur E.: Rules for foot health. J. Practical Nursing, 18:25, May 1968.
Schlosser, Dee: Nursing care of the arthritis patient. J. Practical Nursing, 15:29, May 1965.

ANATOMY AND PHYSIOLOGY REVIEW

1. Label the bones on Figure 43.

   A. Clavicle
   B. Humerus
   C. Radius
   D. Ulna
   E. Sternum
   F. Femur
   G. Patella
   H. Tibia
   I. Fibula
   J. Vertebrae
   K. Pelvis
   L. Phalanges
   M. Metacarpals
   N. Ribs
   O. Cranium

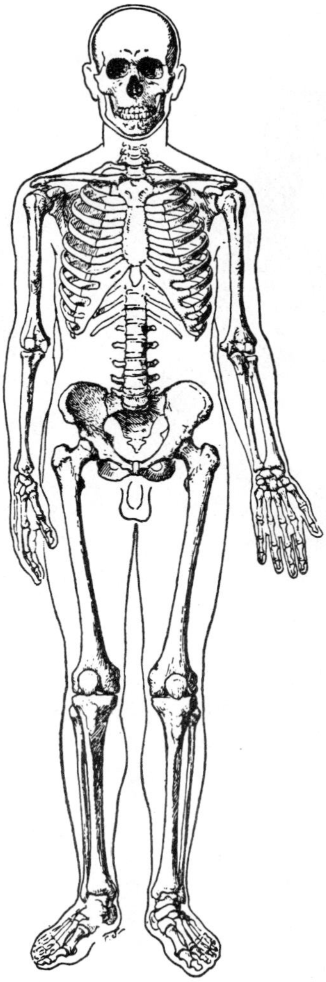

Fig. 43. The skeleton, front view. (Jones and Shepard: Manual of Surgical Anatomy.)

2. Label the muscles on Figure 44.

A. Gluteus maximus
B. Quadriceps femoris
C. Gastrocnemius
D. Sternocleidomastoideus
E. Latissimus dorsi
F. Intercostales externi
G. Deltoideus
H. Biceps brachii

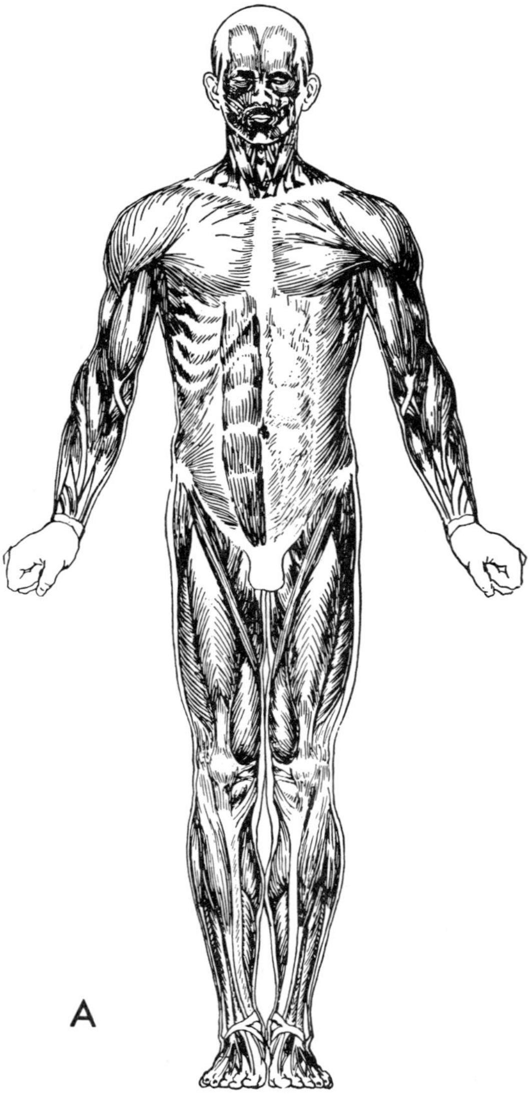

Fig. 44A. Muscles of the body, front view.

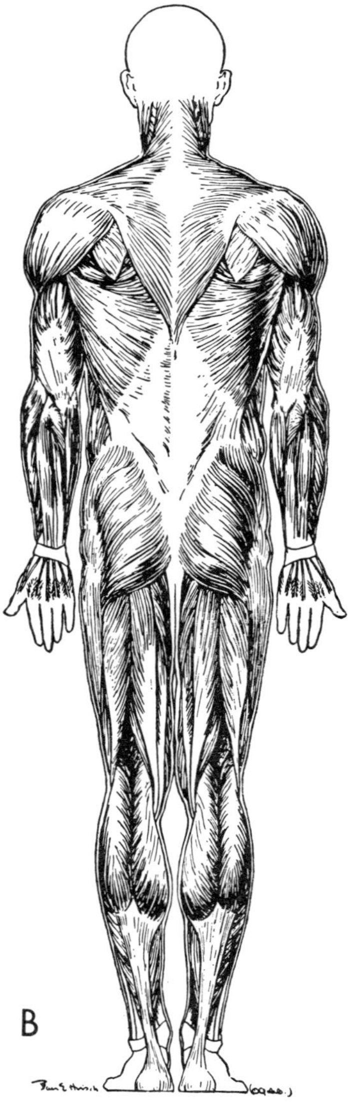

Fig. 44B. Muscles of the body, back view.

(Thompson, E., and LeBaron, M.: Simplified Nursing. 7th ed. Philadelphia, J.B. Lippincott Co., 1960.)

3. Review the terms: flexion, extension, abduction, and adduction.

4. Identify the type movement shown in each figure (Figure 45).

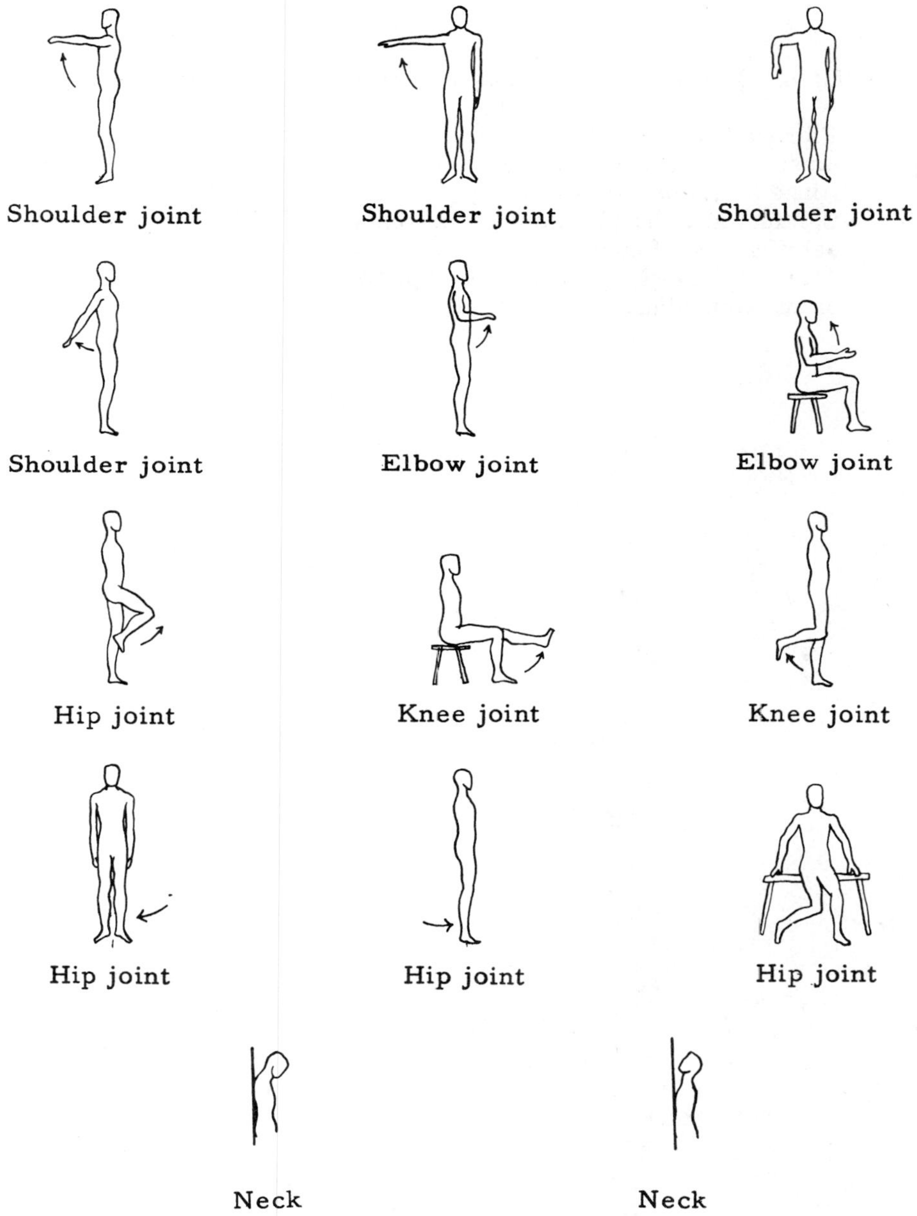

Fig. 45. Joint movements. (McKean, I.: Anatomy and Physiology Laboratory Manual and Study Guide.)

5. What are the functions of

   A. The skeletal system?

   B. The muscular system?

6. True or false. Circle T if the statement is true; F if the statement is false.

T F 1. Fibrous bands which hold bones together are called ligaments.
T F 2. Muscles are attached to bones by fibrous tissue called cartilage.
T F 3. Hinge joints permit a bending motion in only one direction.
T F 4. Calcium and phosphorus must be contained in the diet in order for the calcification of bones to be complete.
T F 5. After prolonged vigorous muscle action, the muscles feel tired because of an accumulation of carbon dioxide.

COMMON ORTHOPEDIC CONDITIONS

1. A fracture is a break in the bone. A simple fracture is a break in a bone in which the ends of the bone do not penetrate the skin. A compound fracture is a broken bone the ends of which penetrate the skin.

A. Draw a greenstick fracture of the femur.

B. Define:

(1) Pathological fracture

(2) Hematoma

C. In what age group does the greenstick fracture usually occur?

D. What effects may a fracture have upon the surrounding tissue?

E. What is the treatment of a fracture?

F. Define:

(1) Closed reduction

(2) Open reduction

2. Osteomyelitis is inflammation of bone. The infection may arise from the entrance of bacteria through an open wound, as in a compound fracture, or it may be an infection carried to the site by the blood from an infected area elsewhere in the body.

A. Symptoms:

B. Treatment:

3. Rickets is a condition caused by an insufficient intake of vitamin D.

A. Symptoms:

B. Treatment:

C. Name two factors which have contributed to the decline of incidence of rickets.

D. Name two excellent sources of vitamin D.

4. Bursitis is inflammation of the bursal sacs of the joints. The joints most commonly involved are the knee, elbow and shoulder.

A. Symptoms:

B. Treatment:

5. A dislocation is a displacement of the bones forming a joint.

A. Symptoms:

B. Treatment:

C. What type of dislocation is commonly a congenital condition?

(1) Symptoms:

(2) Treatment:

(3) Why is an early diagnosis important?

6. Muscular dystrophy is a condition in which certain muscles degenerate and progressively weaken.

A. Cause:

B. Symptoms:

C. Treatment:

7. A sprain is a condition in which a ligament is torn or stretched.

A. Symptoms:

B. Treatment:

8. A sarcoma is a malignant tumor of the bone.

A. Symptoms:

B. Treatment:

9. Arthritis is inflammation of the joints. Arthritis may be acute or chronic. Acute arthritis is usually the result of an infection, trauma or allergy. Acute arthritis commonly occurs as a complication of infections such as rheumatic fever, typhoid fever and lobar pneumonia. Chronic arthritis may also be caused by infectious diseases, such as syphilis and tuberculosis, but the two commonest forms of chronic arthritis are rheumatoid arthritis and hypertrophic arthritis. The causes of these two types of arthritis are unknown.

A. Rheumatoid Arthritis.

(1) List four predisposing factors.

(2) Symptoms:

(3) In what age group does the disease usually occur?

(4) Which joints are most commonly affected?

(5) Medical treatment:

(a) What is the action of aspirin?

(b) Name two hormones used.

(c) Which gland in the body secretes each of these hormones?

(d) What forms of physiotherapy are most commonly used?

(e) What is the difference between active and passive exercise?

(f) What type diet is usually prescribed?

(6) Surgical treatment:

(a) Define:

1. Arthrotomy

2. Arthroplasty

B. Hypertrophic Arthritis.

(1) In what age group does this type of arthritis usually occur?

(2) What is another term for this type of arthritis?

(3) Which joints are most frequently affected?

(4) Treatment:

GENERAL NURSING CARE

1. Multiple Choice.

Mary Ann, age eighteen months, was admitted to the hospital for the treatment of a bilateral congenital dislocation of the hip. She was taken to the cast room where a cast was applied covering the body from the waist down and covering both legs to the ankles.

(1) Before applying a cast, the skin may be protected by covering the area with

(a) Stockinette.
(b) Gauze squares.
(c) Muslin bandage.

(2) Before using plaster of Paris bandage, the roll is placed on end in

(a) Alcohol.
(b) Ether.
(c) Warm water.

(3) A cast in itself is a form of

(1) Open reduction.
(2) Closed reduction.

(4) After the cast has been applied, care must be taken in moving Mary Ann while the cast is wet because

(a) There is danger that the part may become swollen.
(b) There is danger of cracking the cast.
(c) It may prevent the fracture from setting properly.

(5) Mary Ann has a bar attached to her cast, the ends of which are fastened to each leg between the knees. The purpose of this bar is to

(a) Serve as a handgrip when moving the patient.
(b) Aid in the removal of the cast.
(c) Strengthen the cast.

(6) The purpose of Mary Ann's cast is to

(a) Immobilize the femur.
(b) Immobilize the vertebral column.
(c) Reduce the fracture.

(7) The practical nurse can best help in preventing the perineal area of the cast from becoming soiled by

(a) Keeping the bedpan within the reach of the patient.
(b) Lining the edges of the cast with oiled silk or a thin changeable pad.
(c) Frequently turning the patient.

(8) Congenital dislocation of the hip means

(a) This is an inherited condition.
(b) The dislocation resulted from an injury at birth.
(c) The condition was present at birth.

(9) Objective symptoms which the nurse should report in Mary Ann's case are

(a) Complaints of a burning sensation under the cast.
(b) Swelling and cyanosis of the toes.
(c) Inability to flex the knees.

(10) Devices used to properly support Mary Ann are

(a) Pillows and sandbags.
(b) Bed cradle and air ring.
(c) None of these.

Mrs. K., age thirty-five, was admitted to the hospital with a diagnosis of rheumatoid arthritis of the right knee. Her orders included: bed rest, high vitamin, high caloric, high iron diet; aspirin grains five q.4h; traction applied to the right leg as shown in Figure 46.

(11) Arthritis is inflammation of the

(a) Muscles.
(b) Bones.
(c) Joints.

(12) The cause of rheumatoid arthritis is

(a) Spirochete.
(b) Virus.
(c) Unknown.

(13) Rheumatoid arthritis usually occurs during

(a) Adolescence.
(b) Middle age.
(c) Old age.

(14) Mrs. K. is often irritable and depressed. This is understandable because patients with arthritis

(a) Are usually mentally ill.
(b) Are often fearful of permanent crippling.
(c) Have a low threshold for pain.

(15) The purpose of traction is to

(a) Pull muscles in a certain direction.
(b) Prevent decubitus ulcers.
(c) Reduce swelling.

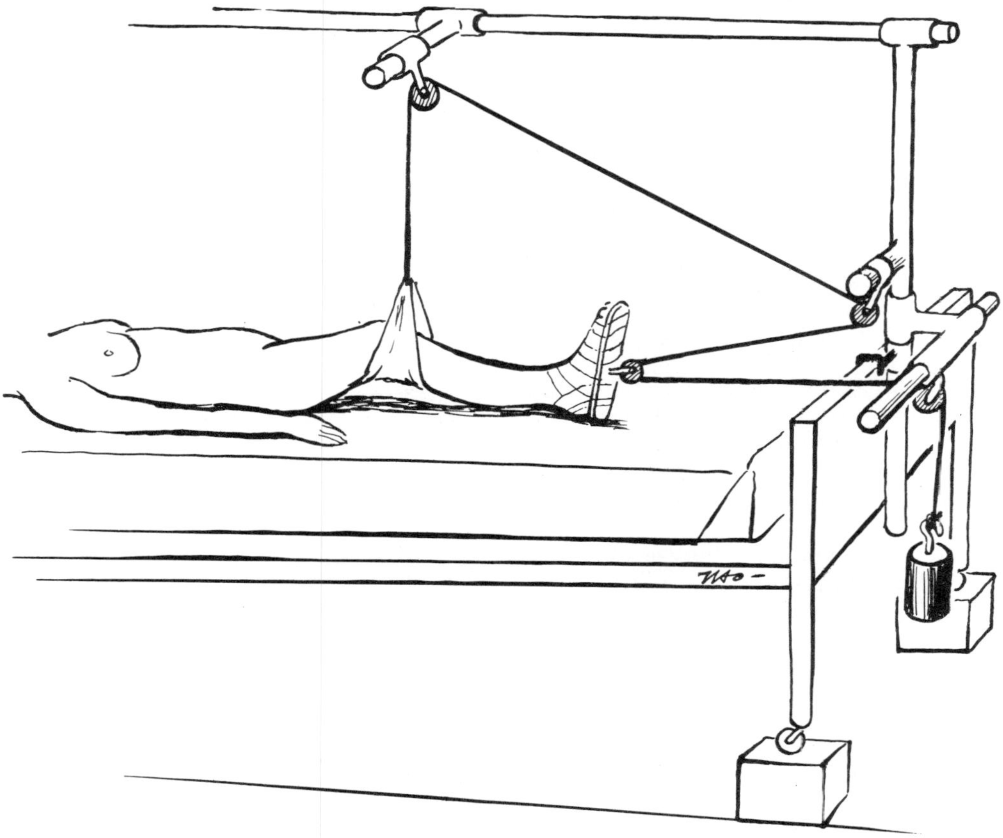

Fig. 46. Patient in traction.

(16) In Figure 46 the purpose of the hammock is to

(a) Pull the muscles of the leg.
(b) Elevate and support the knee.
(c) Abduct the leg.

(17) The foot of the bed is elevated to

(a) Provide countertraction.
(b) Allow for proper support of the leg.
(c) Prevent shock.

(18) Place a check mark in front of each circumstance which would lessen the amount of traction desired in Figure 46.

(a) Weights resting on the floor.
(b) The foot of the affected leg touching the bottom of the bed.
(c) A pillow supporting the calf of the affected leg.
(d) Pulleys not working properly.
(e) The patient's head slightly elevated.

(19) The food listed below which has the highest iron content is

(a) Milk.
(b) Egg.
(c) Peas.

(20) Mrs. K. should receive her aspirin

(a) Four times daily.
(b) Every four hours.
(c) Every four hours when needed.

(21) The practical nurse may remove Mrs. K.'s traction

(a) When it becomes uncomfortable.
(b) During the morning care procedure.
(c) Only when there is a doctor's order.

(22) Cortisone is a hormone secreted by the

(a) Adrenal.
(b) Pituitary.
(c) Thyroid.

(23) ACTH is a hormone secreted by the

(a) Adrenal.
(b) Pituitary.
(c) Gonads.

(24) One of the newer cortisone derivatives used in the treatment of arthritis is called

(a) Neostigmine bromide.
(b) Colchicine.
(c) Meticorten.

(25) Preparation for crutch walking should begin

(a) The first day the patient is allowed out of bed.
(b) After the crutches have been properly fitted.
(c) While the patient is still in bed.

(26) The practical nurse can help in the preparation of the patient for crutch walking by

(a) Demonstrating the use of crutches to the patient.
(b) Making certain that the patient's position always follows the principles of good body alignment.
(c) Removing all obstacles from the floor of the room.

(27) In the four-point-gait method of crutch walking

(a) Weight is partially borne on both legs.
(b) Full weight can be borne on one leg and partial weight on the other.
(c) No weight is borne on either leg.

(28) A replacement for a missing part of the human body is called a

(a) Cosmetic.
(b) Genetic.
(c) Prosthesis.

2. Discussion.

A. List five important aspects of the postoperative care of the amputee.

B. To which agencies in your community might a patient with an orthopedic condition be referred for rehabilitation?

C. What helpful information concerning a prosthetic limb could you give to a patient?

D. How can the nurse be a health teacher in caring for a patient with an orthopedic condition?

E. Discuss the care of braces.

Chapter 36

DISEASES OF THE CIRCULATORY SYSTEM

ANATOMY AND PHYSIOLOGY REVIEW
DIAGNOSTIC PROCEDURES
DISEASE CONDITIONS: CONGENITAL HEART DISEASE, RHEUMATIC HEART DISEASE, CORONARY THROMBOSIS, ARTERIOSCLEROSIS, HYPERTENSION, INFECTIONS, CONGESTIVE HEART FAILURE, VARICOSE VEINS, PHLEBITIS, ANEMIA, LEUKEMIA
GENERAL NURSING CARE

REFERENCES

Culver, V.: Modern Bedside Nursing, Chapters 10 and 46.
Hoffman, C. P., Lipkin, G. P., and Thompson, E. M.: Simplified Nursing, Chapter 32.
Johnston, D. F.: Total Patient Care, Chapter 12.
Keane, C. B.: Essentials of Nursing, Chapter 12.
Mason, M. A.: Basic Medical and Surgical Nursing, Chapters 9-11.
Rapier, D. K., et al.: Practical Nursing, pp. 399-400 and 416-417.
Thompson, E., and Murphy, C.: Textbook of Basic Nursing, Chapter 36.

JOURNALS

Rogoz, Barbara D., and Holswade, George R.: Care of patients having open-heart surgery. J. Practical Nursing, 16:22, April 1966.
The LPN in the intensive care unit. J. Practical Nursing, 16:30, Nov. 1966.

ANATOMY AND PHYSIOLOGY REVIEW

1. Label the parts of the heart (Figure 47).

   A. Right atrium
   B. Left atrium
   C. Right ventricle
   D. Left ventricle
   E. Mitral valve
   F. Tricuspid valve
   G. Pulmonary valve
   H. Aortic valve
   I. Inferior vena cava
   J. Superior vena cava
   K. Aorta
   L. Pulmonary vein
   M. Pulmonary arteries

2. Complete.

   A. The pressure the blood exerts against the walls of the arteries is called ______________________________ .

   B. The rhythmic beating of the heart is called ________________.

   C. The blood platelets aid in __________________ the blood.

   D. The usual amount of blood in the body is ______________________________ .

   E. A substance in the red blood cells which contains iron and carries oxygen is called. ________________________ .

   F. Red blood cells are made in the ___________________________ .

   G. All the arteries but the ___________________ artery carry oxygenated blood.

   H. ______________________ connect the arteries to the veins.

   I. The blood leaves ___________________ in the lungs and picks up ____________________ .

   J. The muscular part of the heart is called _______________________ .

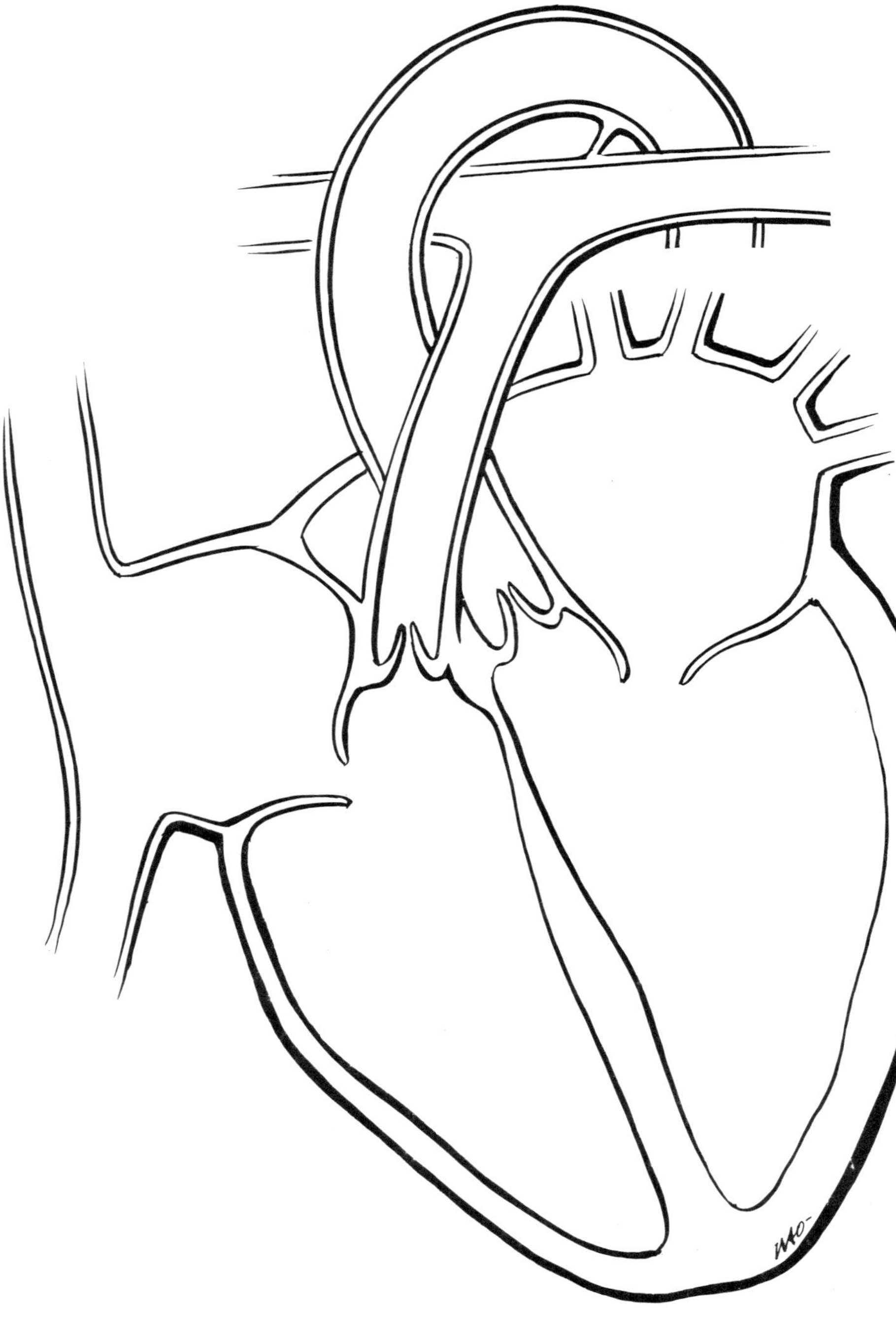

Fig. 47. Heart chambers.

DIAGNOSTIC PROCEDURES

1. Explain the general abnormalities of the circulatory system which may be detected by each of the following diagnostic examinations:

A. X-ray

B. Electrocardiogram

C. Complete blood count

D. Cardiac catheterization

2. List the characteristics of the pulse which should be observed when taking the pulse rate.

DISEASE CONDITIONS

1. Congenital heart disease. There are many variations of congenital defects which may occur in the heart. Two common defects are patent ductus arteriosus and dextrocardia.

A. What is the chief course of treatment for any congenital heart defect?

B. Define hypothermia.

2. Rheumatic heart disease is a complication of rheumatic fever, a disease of children and young adults. Rheumatic fever may cause both an acute and chronic type of heart disease. When rheumatic fever affects the heart, there is an acute inflammation of the entire heart. The inflammation may result in permanent damage to any one of the heart layers. However, the most common result is an inflammation of the endocardium and the formation of lesions which affect the mitral or aortic valve.

A. Define:

(1) Mitral insufficiency

(2) Mitral stenosis

B. What is the treatment for both of these conditions?

C. Do all patients who have rheumatic fever develop rheumatic heart disease?

3. Coronary thrombosis is a condition affecting the coronary arteries, the blood vessels which supply blood to the heart muscle.

A. Define thrombosis.

B. Give symptoms.

C. For what are the symptoms sometimes mistaken?

D. What is the common term for coronary thrombosis?

E. Define infarct.

F. Describe the pain associated with coronary thrombosis?

G. What results if the necrotic heart muscle ruptures?

H. Name a medication used in treating coronary thrombosis that has the action of

(1) Relieving pain.
(2) Preventing a second blood clot from forming.
(3) Dilating the coronary blood vessels.

4. Arteriosclerosis is a disease in which the arteries slowly become hardened.

A. Cause:

B. Symptoms:

C. Complications:

5. Hypertension, or high blood pressure, is a symptom of certain diseases. Hypertension, however, may also be a disease in itself.

A. Cause:

B. Symptoms:

C. Complications:

D. Treatment:

6. Infections may occur in the heart and cause permanent damage. The organisms most frequently causing heart infection are streptococcus, pneumococcus and gonococcus. These infections may be either acute or subacute.

A. Define subacute.

B. What is the term used to describe an inflammation of the

(1) Endocardium?
(2) Pericardium?
(3) Myocardium?

C. Which group of medications has greatly reduced the fatality rate of heart infections?

D. In what way does a subacute bacterial endocarditis usually damage the heart?

7. Congestive heart failure is really a complication of other types of heart disease; it may occur in any heart disease. The symptoms of congestive heart failure arise from the fact that the heart is unable to function properly as a pump. In the early stages of heart failure the symptoms are moderate. In the advanced stages all of the early symptoms are greatly aggravated.

A. Symptoms:

B. Treatment:

(1) Why may each of the following types of medication be necessary?

(a) Analgesic

(b) Diuretic

(c) Sedative

(d) Mild laxative

(e) Oxygen therapy

(2) Define:

(a) Abdominal paracentesis

(b) Thoracentesis

(3) What methods are used to measure the amount of body fluid loss per day?

(4) Discuss the diet restrictions and give the reasons why these restrictions are needed.

8. Varicose veins is a condition affecting the valves of the veins and causing an interference in the flow of blood from the small veins into the larger veins in the return flow of blood to the heart.

A. Predisposing factors:

B. Prevention:

C. Symptoms:

D. What is the term used to describe the surgical treatment?

E. Medical treatment:

F. What is the term for varicose veins of the rectum?

9. Phlebitis is inflammation of a vein. The inflammation usually causes a thrombus to form in the vein. It is possible, however, for a blood clot to form in the vein without the presence of an inflammation. The symptoms resulting from both of these abnormalities are somewhat the same.

A. What is the lay term for phlebitis of the leg?

B. Predisposing factors:

C. Symptoms:

D. Medical treatment:

E. Surgical treatment:

10. Anemia is a decrease in the normal amount of hemoglobin in the blood.

A. Cause:

B. Symptoms:

C. Treatment:

11. Leukemia is malignant disease of the blood in which the white blood cells destroy the red blood cells. There are several types of leukemia which are classified according to the type of white blood cell which predominantly increases in number. What are the two main types of white blood cells?

GENERAL NURSING CARE

A. Match each medication commonly used in treating circulatory diseases with the the correct action.

Medication		Action
a. Dicumarol	______	1. Vasodilator
b. Adrenalin	______	2. Lowers the blood pressure
c. Nitroglycerin	______	3. Analgesic
d. Mercuhydrin	______	4. Anticoagulant
e. Resperine	______	5. Antianemic
f. Digitalis	______	6. Emergency stimulant
g. Demerol	______	7. Sedative
h. Penicillin	______	8. Diuretic
i. Liver extract	______	9. Slows and strengthens the heart beat
j. Phenobarbital	______	10. Antibiotic

B. Match each medication with the correct signs of overdosage.

Medication		Signs of Overdosage
a. Digitalis	______	1. Hematuria
b. Morphine	______	2. Headaches, faintness, heart palpitations
c. Dicumarol	______	3. Slow respirations, pin-point pupils, comatose sleep
d. Aspirin	______	4. Hives, swelling of the skin and mucous membranes
e. Quinidine	______	5. Slowing of the heart rate, nausea

C. Multiple Choice. Circle the letter preceding the correct answer to each statement.

Mrs. J., age fifty-five, was admitted to the hospital with a diagnosis of congestive heart failure. Her symptoms were severe dyspnea, an irregular rapid pulse, edema of both legs and cyanosis of the lips.

(1) The term dyspnea means

(a) Rapid pulse.
(b) Difficult respirations.
(c) Difficulty in voiding.

(2) When a patient can breathe only while sitting, the condition is called

(a) Cheyne-Stokes respirations.
(b) Apnea.
(c) Orthopnea.

(3) Cyanosis is caused by a

(a) Deficiency of iron in the blood.
(b) Lack of red blood cells.
(c) Deficient amount of oxygen in the blood.

(4) Mrs. J.'s edema is caused by

(a) An accumulation of fluid in the tissues due to poor circulation.
(b) An inflammation of the tissues.
(c) Lack of exercise.

(5) On admission Mrs. J. was placed in bed. Her backrest was elevated to an upright position and her knees were slightly flexed. This position is called

(a) Semi-Fowler's.
(b) Fowler's.
(c) Dorsal recumbent.

(6) Another position which would help to relieve Mrs. J.'s dyspnea is

(a) Turning the patient on her side.
(b) Placing pillows on an over-bed table and allowing the patient to lean forward on it.
(c) Having the patient sit on the side of the bed.

Mrs. J.'s orders include a low sodium diet; complete bed rest; digitalis gr. $\overline{\text{iss}}$ t.i.d.; Nembutal gr. $\overline{\text{iss}}$ h.s.p.r.n. and nasal oxygen administered at a flow of five liters per minute.

(7) Circle the letter preceding each statement which is true concerning a low sodium diet.

(a) Foods may be cooked with a small amount of salt.
(b) No salt is allowed at the table.
(c) Milk is allowed.
(d) Ice cream is to be avoided.
(e) All types of regular bread are allowed.
(f) All foods prepared with baking powder and baking soda are to be avoided.
(g) Unsalted butter is used.
(h) There is no substitute for the salt seasoning

(8) The approximate percentage of sodium contained in salt is

(a) 5.
(b) 15.
(c) 40.

(9) In giving Mrs. J. morning care, the nurse will be responsible for

(a) Generally assisting with the bath and oral hygiene; serving breakfast and making an occupied bed.
(b) Lifting and moving the patient; giving a complete bed bath; brushing the patient's teeth; feeding the patient and making an occupied bed.
(c) Assisting with the bath and oral hygiene; feeding the patient; assisting the patient in getting out of bed and making an unoccupied bed.

(10) Before administering the digitalis, the nurse should check Mrs. J's

(a) Temperature, pulse and respiration.
(b) Respiration and pulse
(c) Pulse only.

(11) Digitalis should not be given if

(a) The respirations are above 20 per minute.
(b) The pulse rate is below 60 beats per minute.
(c) Both of these conditions exist.

(12) The nurse should administer the digitalis as follows:

(a) Grams 1-1/2 twice daily.
(b) Grams 1-1/2 three times daily.
(c) Grains 1-1/2 three times daily.

(13) In giving nasal oxygen, the tip of the nasal catheter should be located in the

(a) Pharynx.
(b) Larynx.
(c) Trachea.

(14) Circle the number preceding each statement which is true concerning the care of the patient receiving nasal oxygen therapy.

(a) No smoking should be permitted in the patient's room.
(b) The oxygen must be humidified.
(c) The nasal catheter should be changed no oftener than every three days.
(d) The patient's nares should be kept well lubricated to prevent irritation.
(e) The nasal catheter should be taped to the patient's face.

(15) Nembutal is

(a) An opiate.
(b) A barbiturate.
(c) An anesthetic.

(16) In order to prevent a decubitus ulcer, skin care is especially important for the cardiac patient because

(a) Most cardiac patients are elderly.
(b) There is circulatory impairment.
(c) The skin usually becomes dry.

(17) Heart disease is

(a) The leading cause of deaths.
(b) The second leading cause of deaths.
(c) The third leading cause of deaths.

(18) An accumulation of fluids in the abdomen is called

(a) Ascites.
(b) Peritonitis.
(c) Paracentesis.

(19) In giving a cardiac patient an enema, the nurse would

(a) Use a smaller amount of solution than usual.
(b) Place the patient on the right side instead of the left.
(c) Give it with the patient sitting on a commode.

D. Discuss the socioeconomic aspects of heart disease.

E. Is there a branch office of the American Heart Association in your community? If so, where is it located?

F. What other agencies in your community may be of some assistance to the patient who is discharged from the hospital as a "cardiac cripple"?

Chapter 37

DISEASES OF THE RESPIRATORY SYSTEM

ANATOMY AND PHYSIOLOGY REVIEW
DIAGNOSTIC PROCEDURES
DISEASE CONDITIONS: COMMON COLD, TONSILLITIS, LARYNGITIS, BRONCHITIS, BRONCHIECTASIS, PNEUMONIA, ALLERGIES, PULMONARY TUBERCULOSIS
GENERAL NURSING CARE

REFERENCES

Culver, V.: Modern Bedside Nursing, Chapters 9 and 45.
Hoffman, C. P., Lipkin, G. P., and Thompson, E. M.: Simplified Nursing, Chapter 33.
Johnston, D. F.: Total Patient Care, Chapter 10.
Keane, C. B.: Essentials of Nursing, Chapter 13.
Mason, M. A.: Basic Medical and Surgical Nursing, Chapters 12 and 13.
Rapier, D. K., et al.: Practical Nursing, pp. 405-407.
Thompson, E., and Murphy, C.: Textbook of Basic Nursing, Chapter 39.

JOURNALS

Day, Faye G.: Cystic fibrosis – a serious lung condition of children. Am. J. Practical Nursing, 1:102, Sept. 1965.
Fahy, Agnes: The LPN and the care of the tuberculosis patient. Am. J. Practical Nursing, 2:9, Jan. 1966.
Fontana, Vincent J., and Rappaport, Irwin: Asthma. J. Practical Nursing, 15:24, Dec. 1965.
Rehabilitation of emphysema and chronic bronchitis patients. Bedside Nurse, 1:23, March-April 1969.

ANATOMY AND PHYSIOLOGY REVIEW

1. Color the parts of the respiratory system in Figure 48.

   A. Trachea - yellow
   B. Larynx - red
   C. Bronchi - blue

2. Label the parts.

   A. Bronchiole
   B. Alveoli

3. Complete.

   A. As air enters the nasal passage, it is cleaned and warmed.

   B. The roof of the mouth is called the palate.

   C. The cavities in the bones of the skull are called paranasal sinus. The total number of these is four.

   D. The Adam's apple is part of the thyroid cartilage & ~~larynx~~ larynx

   E. The twofold function of the larynx is that of passageway and voice box speech.

   F. The left lung has 2 lobes; the right lung 3 lobes.

   G. The respiratory center of the brain is located in the medulla or cerebral cortex

   H. The movements of respiration are controlled by the action of the diaphragm and intercostal muscles.

   I. In the exchange of gases in the lungs, the blood cells pick up O_2 and leave CO_2.

   J. The body cells need oxygen for oxidation of foodstuffs to produce heat.

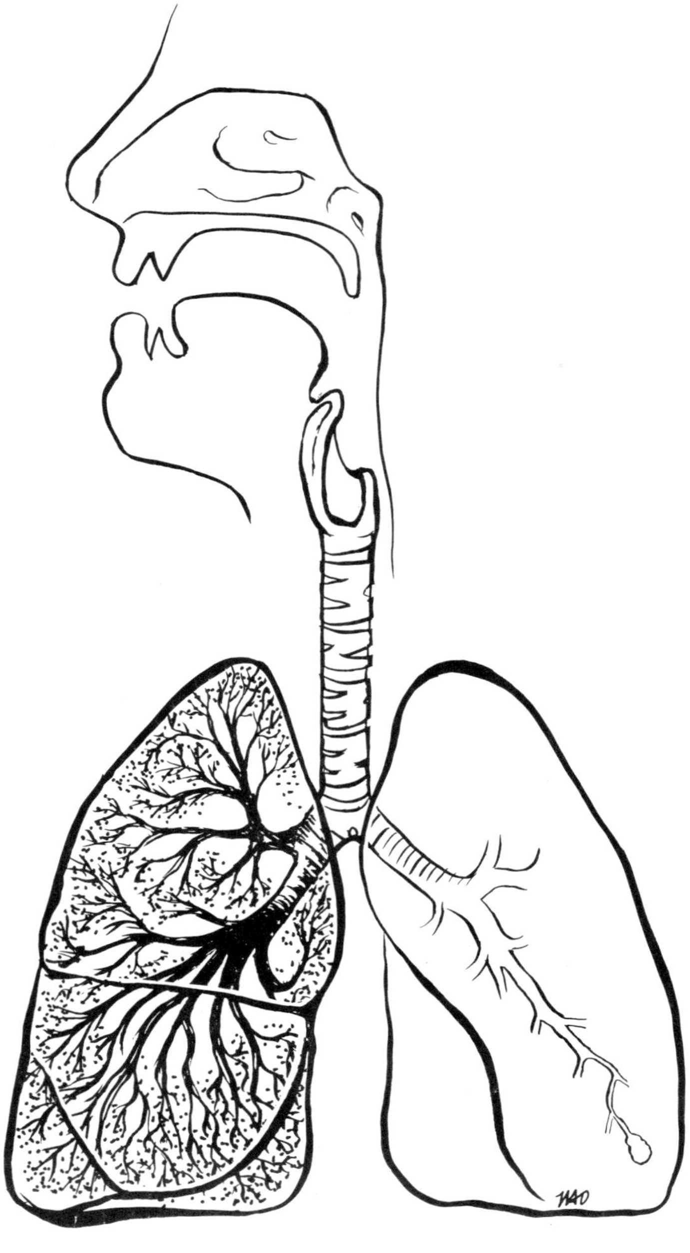

Fig. 48. Respiratory system.

DIAGNOSTIC PROCEDURES

Complete the table.

DIAGNOSTIC PROCEDURE	DEFINITION	PREPARATION OF PATIENT	PRACTICAL NURSE RESPONSIBILITIES
Bronchogram			
Bronchoscopy			
Chest x-ray			

COMMON DISEASE CONDITIONS

1. The common cold, or coryza, is inflammation of the mucous lining of the nasal passage.

A. Predisposing factors:

B. Cause:

C. Symptoms:

D. Treatment:

E. Complications:

F. Preventive measures:

G. Economic problems:

2. Tonsillitis is inflammation of the tonsils, usually caused by a streptococcus.

A. Symptoms:

B. Treatment:

3. Laryngitis is inflammation of the larynx. It may arise as a complication of the common cold or it may follow the improper use of the voice.

A. Symptoms:

B. Treatment:

C. What is croup?

D. In what age group does croup usually occur?

4. Bronchitis is inflammation of the bronchial tubes. It may be either acute or chronic.

A. Symptoms:

B. Treatment:

5. Bronchiectasis is a chronic disease of the bronchial tubes in which one or more of the tubes dilate.

A. Symptoms:

B. Treatment:

C. What nursing measures can be carried out to improve the appetite of a patient who coughs up large amounts of foul-tasting and foul-smelling sputum?

6. Pneumonia is inflammation of the lung. There are several types of pneumonia which may be either acute or chronic.

A. Causative organisms:

B. Discuss the variation of the symptoms in

(1) Bronchopneumonia

(2) Lobar pneumonia

(3) Virus pneumonia

C. Treatment:

7. Certain conditions of the respiratory system are due to allergies. Hay fever is a condition that results from the inhalation of allergens or substances to which the body is hypersensitive. Hay fever may be seasonal (due to the inhalation of pollen from plants) or it may occur the year round (due to the inhalation of dust, etc.). Bronchial asthma is a condition which affects the mucous lining of the bronchial tubes. Asthma may also be seasonal or nonseasonal and usually is caused by the same allergens that cause hay fever. In addition, food allergy is a frequent cause of bronchial asthma.

A. What is a sensitivity test?

B. How can one tell if a sensitivity test is positive?

C. Complete the table.

	SYMPTOMS	TREATMENT
Hay fever		
Asthma		

D. Explain the action of each medication.

(1) Adrenalin

(2) Isuprel

(3) Aminophylline

(4) Ephedrine

E. Name two antihistaminic drugs.

8. Pulmonary tuberculosis is an infectious disease which causes more deaths than any other infectious disease. Tuberculosis may involve almost any organ of the body but occurs principally in the lung.

A. Causative organism:

B. Ways of contracting the disease:

C. Preventive measures:

D. Age group most susceptible:

E. Symptoms:

F. Medical treatment:

G. Surgical treatment:

GENERAL NURSING CARE

1. Practical Nurse E. accepted a home nursing case. The patient, Mrs. M., age forty-one, had an upper respiratory infection. She complained of nasal congestion, headache, malaise, nasal discharge and sore throat. Her orders included: saline gargle b.i.d.; Crysticillin 300,000 U. I.M., at 10:00 A.M. daily; steam inhalations one-half hour t.i.d.; soft diet; bed rest with bathroom privileges; and aspirin gr. x p.r.n. for headache.

A. The upper respiratory tract includes the

(1) Nose, throat and sinuses.
(2) Nose, throat, sinuses and larynx.
(3) Nose, throat, sinuses, larynx and trachea.

B. Nasal congestion is caused by

(1) The swelling of the mucous membranes of the nasal passages.
(2) Increased secretions.
(3) Neither of these.

C. The term malaise means

(1) Breathing through the mouth.
(2) A generalized feeling of discomfort.
(3) Swelling of the neck glands.

D. To prepare the solution for the saline gargle, the practical nurse correctly mixed

(1) One teaspoon of salt in one quart of tap water.
(2) One teaspoon of salt in one pint of tap water.
(3) One tablespoon of salt in one pint of tap water.

E. The temperature of the solution for a throat gargle should be

(1) 90 to 100 degrees Fahrenheit.
(2) 100 to 110 degrees Fahrenheit.
(3) 110 to 120 degrees Fahrenheit.

F. The action of Crysticillin is

(1) Antibiotic.
(2) Antidote.
(3) Antipruritic.

G. When giving the injection, the syringe should be held at what angle to the body?

(1) 15 degrees.
(2) 45 degrees.
(3) 90 degrees.

H. Mrs. M. does not have a steam inhalator. Practical Nurse E. should

(1) Explain to the patient that it will be necessary to purchase an inhalator at the drug store.
(2) Place a teakettle of water on the stove, attach a newspaper funnel and request the patient to go to the kitchen for the treatment.
(3) Place a pitcher of very hot water at the patient's bedside and direct the flow of steam toward the patient by placing a paper bag with a hole in it over the pitcher.

I. A medication sometimes ordered by the physician to be used in the steam inhalation is

(1) Tincture of benzoin.
(2) Benzedrine sulfate.
(3) Benzyl benzoate.

J. After the steam inhalation treatment, the practical nurse should

(1) Place the patient in Fowler's position for a short period of time.
(2) Keep the patient warm and avoid drafts to prevent chills.
(3) Request the patient to cough so that the bronchial secretions will be loosened.

K. In suggesting a luncheon menu for Mrs. M., the practical nurse mentioned

(1) Frankfurter on toasted bun, tossed salad, ice cream and tea.
(2) Tomato juice, creamed chicken on toast, canned peaches and coffee.
(3) Poached egg on toast, carrot sticks, strawberries and milk.

L. The aspirin on hand contains five grains per tablet. Mrs. M. should be given

(1) One tablet.
(2) One-half tablet.
(3) Two tablets.

M. Circle the number preceding each nursing procedure which is necessary in maintaining medical asepsis in the care of Mrs. M.

(1) Pinning a paper bag on the side of the bed to be used as a receptacle for soiled tissues.
(2) Instructing the patient in the proper use of tissues.
(3) Disinfecting the excreta.
(4) Boiling the dishes after use.
(5) Burning the soiled tissues.

2. The purpose of artificial pneumothorax in the treatment of pulmonary tuberculosis is to

A. Remove fluid from the thoracic cavity.
B. Collapse all or part of the affected lung so that it may heal while at rest.
C. Remove the affected lung.

3. Postural drainage is a treatment used to allow for the drainage of suppurative material from the lung. The drainage is made possible by

A. The force of gravity.
B. The use of a suction apparatus.
C. An aspirating machine.

4. An important point for the practical nurse to remember when encountering a closed chest drainage apparatus is that

A. The apparatus must always be kept airtight.
B. She should refuse to perform any act of nursing care for a patient with closed chest drainage.
C. The care of the apparatus is usually the responsibility of the physician.

5. Coughing up blood or blood-streaked sputum is called

A. Hemoptysis.
B. Hematemesis.
C. Hematoma.

6. The normal percentage of oxygen in the air is

A. 10 per cent.
B. 15 per cent.
C. 20 per cent.

7. When administering oxygen therapeutically, the approximate percentage of oxygen concentration needed in the air the patient is inhaling is

A. 20 per cent.
B. 50 per cent.
C. 100 per cent.

8. When a patient is receiving oxygen in a tent, certain precautions such as substituting a hand bell for an electric call bell and using cotton instead of wool blankets are necessary because

A. The tent is usually made of an inflammable material.
B. They help to increase the oxygen concentration in the tent.
C. Oxygen supports combustion.

9. The best type of container to use for collecting a sputum specimen is one which can be

A. Burned after use.
B. Boiled after use.
C. Autoclaved after use.

10. The best way to help lessen the fears of the patient with a tracheotomy tube is to

A. Keep the patient in a semi-Fowler's position.
B. Teach the patient as much as possible concerning the care of the tube.
C. Make certain the patient has a call bell.

11. In caring for a patient with a tracheotomy tube, the main object in the care of the tube is to

A. Prevent the tube from becoming obstructed with mucus.
B. Prevent tarnishing of the tube.
C. Prevent denting of the tube.

12. A medication given with oxygen to aid in loosening respiratory secretions is

A. Alevaire.
B. Alidase.
C. Aminophylline.

13. The tubercle bacillus was discovered by

A. Robert Koch.
B. Louis Pasteur.
C. Charles Mantoux.

14. Two drugs being used effectively in the treatment of tuberculosis are

A. Penicillin and streptomycin.
B. Acetosalicylic acid and cortisone.
C. Para-aminosalicylic acid and isoniazid.

15. Concentrated effort must be given to the diversional therapy program for the convalescent tuberculosis patient because

A. He must continue to restrain his activity even though he feels well.
B. He usually feels too ill to participate in any activity.
C. He is not allowed to have visitors.

Chapter 38

DISEASES OF THE URINARY SYSTEM

ANATOMY AND PHYSIOLOGY REVIEW
DIAGNOSTIC PROCEDURES
DISEASE CONDITIONS: CYSTITIS, NEPHRITIS, PYELITIS, CALCULI, URETHRITIS, NEPHROSIS,
GENERAL NURSING CARE

REFERENCES

Culver, V.: Modern Bedside Nursing, Chapters 13 and 47.
Hoffman, C. P., Lipkin, G. P., and Thompson, E. M.: Simplified Nursing, Chapter 35.
Johnston, D. F.: Total Patient Care, Chapter 14.
Keane, C. B.: Essentials of Nursing, Chapter 15.
Mason, M. A.: Basic Medical and Surgical Nursing, Chapter 19.
Rapier, D. K., et al.: Practical Nursing, pp. 413-416.
Thompson, E., and Murphy, C.: Textbook of Basic Nursing, Chapter 40.

ANATOMY AND PHYSIOLOGY REVIEW

1. In the space provided, draw and label the parts of the urinary system.

2. Complete.

   A. The function of the kidneys is ____.

   B. Urine is secreted by the ____________________.

   C. The male urethra is ___________ inches long; the female urethra is _______ inches long.

   D. The bladder normally can hold ___________ cc. of urine.

   E. The normal daily output of urine is ___________ cc.; however, the output may be influenced by such factors as ____
   ____
   ____.

DIAGNOSTIC PROCEDURES

1. How is the patient prepared for each of the following diagnostic procedures?

   A. Twenty-four hour urine specimen

   B. Intravenous pyelogram

   C. Cystoscopic examination

   D. Phenosulfonphthalein test

   E. Urea clearance

2. How is a sterile urine specimen obtained from

   A. A male patient?

   B. A female patient?

3. How should a urine specimen be correctly labeled in your hospital?

4. How much urine is needed for a single specimen of urine?

COMMON DISEASE CONDITIONS

1. Cystitis is inflammation of the bladder caused by a bacterial infection.

   A. Causative organisms:

   B. Route of entry of the infection:

   C. Symptoms:

   D. Treatment:

2. Nephritis is inflammation of the kidney which causes an impairment of function. This condition usually follows an infection of the upper respiratory tract, especially those infections caused by the hemolytic streptococcus. Nephrisit, formerly called Bright's disease, takes many forms and may be either acute or chronic. The acute form is more common in children than in adults and occurs twice as frequently in males. Chronic nephritis usually occurs in the later years of life. The prognosis for acute nephritis is good, especially in children. However, if the patient does not completely recover from acute nephritis, the chronic form may develop. The prognosis for chronic nephritis is poor.

   A. Complete the table.

NEPHRITIS	SYMPTOMS	TREATMENT
Acute		
Chronic		

   B. How does the edema in nephritis differ from the edema in heart disease?

C. Define uremia.

D. What are the symptoms of uremia?

E. What is the purpose of the Kempner rice diet?

F. Describe the artificial kidney.

3. Pyelitis is inflammation of the kidney pelvis. The infection is usually caused by bacteria which enter the urethra and travel upward to the kidney. Pyelitis seldom causes an impairment in the function of the kidney.

A. Symptoms:

B. Treatment:

4. Calculi, or stones, may form in the kidneys, ureters or bladder. The stones vary in size and may or may not cause distress. Often, however, a small stone may attempt to pass from the pelvis of the kidney through the ureter. This may obstruct the ureter and cause excruciating pains. This pain is called renal and ureteral colic.

A. What changes would occur in the kidney if the ureter were completely obstructed by a stone for a prolonged period of time?

B. Describe the method of straining urine.

5. Urethritis, inflammation of the urethra, is usually caused by the gonococcus.

A. Name the preventive measures promoted by the public health service.

B. Methods of contraction:

C. Symptoms:

D. Treatment:

E. Prognosis:

6. Nephrosis is a condition characterized by a degeneration of the tubules of the kidney. There is no inflammation of the kidney, but the disease may accompany certain infectious diseases. Nephrosis may also result from being transfused with incompatible blood, and it may also be caused by an insufficient fluid intake as during episodes of excessive vomiting and diarrhea. One form of the disease occurs in children and is characterized by severe edema.

A. Treatment:

B. Discuss your understanding of the terms hemodialysis and peritoneal dialysis.

GENERAL NURSING CARE

Multiple Choice. Circle the letter preceding the correct answer to each statement.

Mr. J., age thirty-five, was admitted to the hospital with a diagnosis of acute nephritis.

1. It is very likely that Mr. J.

   A. Recently recovered from an upper respiratory infection.
   B. Has gonorrhea.
   C. Practices poor health habits.

2. The symptoms one would expect Mr. J. to have

   A. Are edema and hypertension.
   B. May be few or numerous since the symptoms of this condition are not the same in every case.
   C. Are usually not discovered until chemical tests of the patient's blood are made.

3. In selecting a semi-private room for Mr. J., you would not place him in a room with a patient who has a diagnosis of

   A. Bronchitis.
   B. Peptic ulcer.
   C. Hypertension.

4. The treatment of nephritis varies, but the one treatment which is given to all patients with nephritis is

   A. The restriction of fluids.
   B. The Kempner rice diet.
   C. Bed rest.

5. Rice contains large quantities of the food nutrient

   A. Ascorbic acid.
   B. Thiamine.
   C. Fat.

6. Mr. J. was to be weighed daily in order to check the amount of fluid loss from the body. An essential in determining an accurate daily weight is to

   A. Weigh the patient at the same time daily.
   B. Remove all clothes from the patient before weighing.
   C. Weigh the patient after the morning bath.

7. Which of the following drugs used in treating urinary diseases is a diuretic?

   A. Gantrisin.
   B. Mandelic acid.
   C. Salyrgan.

8. Which of the following fruits has the highest sodium content?

   A. Dates.
   B. Oranges.
   C. Cherries.

9. Urea frost, a manifestation of uremia, is

   A. The formation of crystals in the urine.
   B. The deposit of a white crystal-like substance on the skin.
   C. A condition in which the skin feels cold to the touch.

10. Mr. E. was admitted to the hospital and an indwelling catheter was put in place. This means

    A. The patient was catheterized in order to obtain a sterile specimen of urine.
    B. The catheter was inserted into the bladder for continuous drainage of urine.
    C. The bladder was irrigated.

11. Figure 49 illustrates the Foley catheter which was inserted into Mr. E's bladder. After the catheter was inserted, the bag, A, was inflated by injecting a sterile solution into

    A. C
    B. A
    C. B

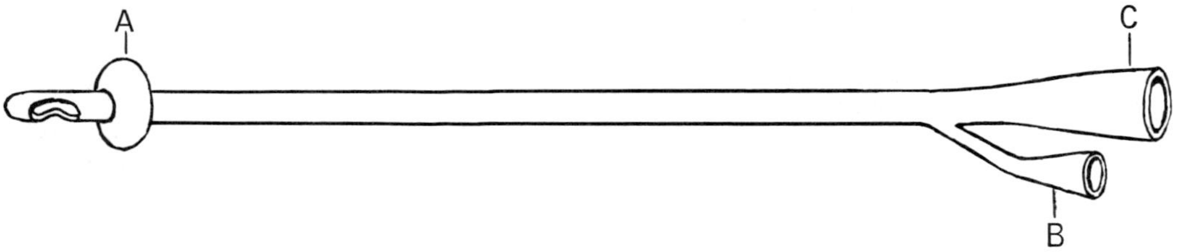

Fig. 49. Foley catheter.

12. The catheter was connected to a drainage tube with a glass connecting tube which was pushed into

    A. C
    B. B
    C. A

13. An order was written to irrigate Mr. E.'s catheter. In irrigating the catheter, the maximum amount of sterile solution to be instilled into the bladder at one time is

A. 25 cc.
B. 100 cc.
C. 200 cc.

14. Mr. E. was on intake and output. In computing the total intake for twenty-four hours, the nurse includes

A. Intravenous fluids, blood transfusions and all fluids taken orally.
B. The oral intake of fluids only.
C. Intravenous fluids and fluids taken orally.

15. After the indwelling catheter was removed from the patient, the nurse was careful to observe for

A. Orchitis.
B. Hematuria.
C. Retention of urine.

16. When urine is not being produced by the kidneys in a sufficient amount, the condition is called

A. Suppression.
B. Retention.
C. Polyuria.

Medication Review. Match each medication with its action.

Action	Medication
a. Antibiotic	_____ 1. Potassium citrate
b. Increases urine acidity	_____ 2. Diamox
c. Makes urine alkaline	_____ 3. Mandelic acid
d. Diuretic	_____ 4. Theobromine
	_____ 5. Gantrisin
	_____ 6. Mercuhydrin
	_____ 7. Esidrix
	_____ 8. Sodium acid phosphate
	_____ 9. Salyrgan
	_____ 10. Streptomycin

Chapter 39

DISEASES OF THE ENDOCRINE SYSTEM

ANATOMY AND PHYSIOLOGY REVIEW
DISEASE CONDITIONS: DISTURBANCES OF THE PITUITARY, PARATHYROID, ADRENAL, GONADS, THYROID; DIABETES MELLITUS
GENERAL NURSING CARE

REFERENCES

Culver, V.: Modern Bedside Nursing, Chapters 14 and 44.
Hoffman, C. P., Lipkin, G. P., and Thompson, E. M.: Simplified Nursing, Chapter 37.
Johnston, D. F.: Total Patient Care, Chapter 16.
Keane, C. B.: Essentials of Nursing, Chapter 16.
Mason, M. A.: Basic Medical and Surgical Nursing, Chapter 18.
Rapier, D. K., et al.: Practical Nursing, pp. 417-422.
Thompson, E., and Murphy, C.: Textbook of Basic Nursing, Chapter 42.

JOURNALS

Martin, Marguerite M.: Foot disorders in diabetes. J. Practical Nursing, 17:32, April 1967.
Martin, Marguerite M.: Insulin, the life-giving hormone. J. Practical Nursing, 18:42, March 1968; 25, April 1968.

ANATOMY AND PHYSIOLOGY REVIEW

1. Draw and label the endocrine glands in Figure 51.

   A. Pituitary
   B. Parathyroid
   C. Thyroid
   D. Thymus
   E. Adrenal
   F. Pancreas
   G. Testis
   H. Ovary

2. Match each endocrine gland with the correct function.

Gland		Function
a. Pituitary	____	1. Controls the rate of the vital processes of the body
b. Adrenal	____	2. Controls the metabolism of the carbohydrates
c. Thyroid	____	3. Regulate the secondary sex characteristics
d. Gonads	____	4. Aids the body in emergency stress situations
e. Pancreas	____	5. Aids in controlling all of the endocrine glands

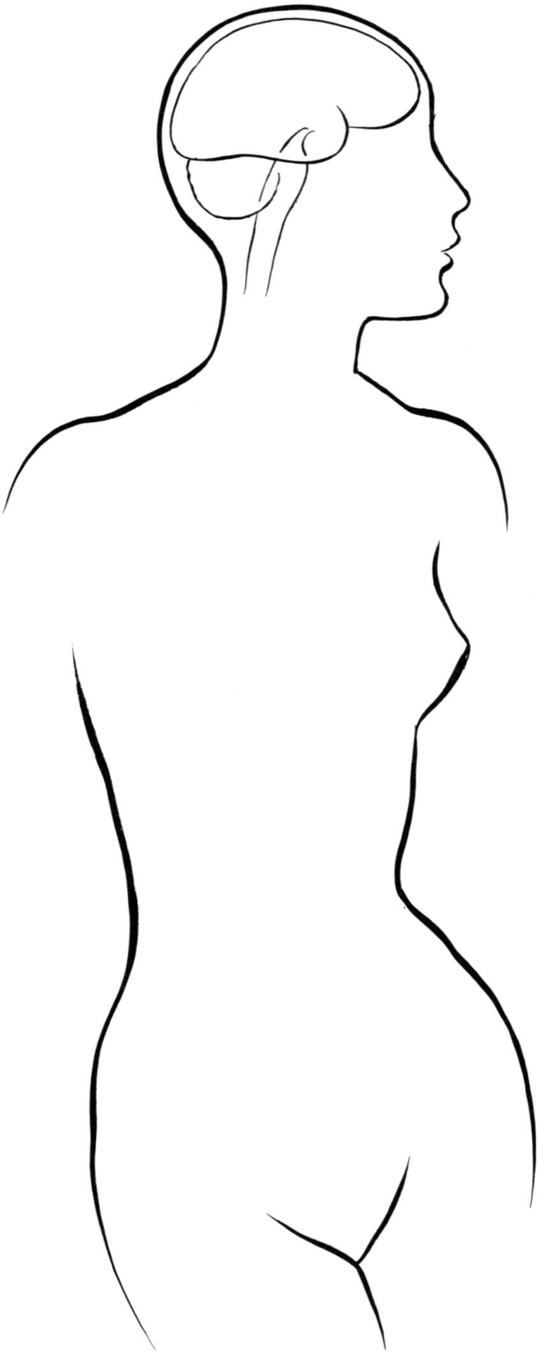

Fig. 50. Outline of the body.

DISEASE CONDITIONS

1. Complete the table.

GLAND	CONDITION RESULTING FROM HYPERFUNCTION	CONDITION RESULTING FROM HYPOFUNCTION
Pituitary		
Parathyroid		
Adrenal		
Gonads		

2. Thyroid Disturbances. The abnormalities of the thyroid gland result from hyperactivity, hypoactivity, a deficiency in the intake of iodine or an enlargement of the gland. A deficiency in the iodine intake causes colloid goiter, an enlargement of the gland without a disturbance in function, which usually occurs at the age of puberty. The treatment for colloid goiter is the administration of iodine. If hypoactivity of the thyroid is congenital, it causes a condition known as cretinism; if it occurs in adulthood, the condition is known as myxedema. The treatment for hypoactivity of the thyroid is the oral administration of the thyroid hormone. An enlargement of the thyroid gland associated with a hyperactivity in function results in a condition known as exophthalmic goiter, or Graves' disease. The exact cause is unknown; however, a nervous temperament seems to be a predisposing factor. The condition usually occurs among young adults and affects more women than men.

A. What are the symptoms of cretinism?

B. How is a patient properly prepared for a basal metabolism test?

C. How would you describe the basal metabolism test to the patient?

D. When the radioactive iodine uptake test is done on the patient, what precautions are necessary to protect the nurse from radioactive exposure?

E. List the symptoms of exophthalmic goiter.

F. How can one provide for mental rest in caring for a patient with exophthalmic goiter?

G. Persons suffering from exophthalmic goiter usually require twice the average daily caloric intake and yet there is no weight gain. Why is this true?

H. The treatment of this condition consists of the administration of Lugol's solution, a compound solution of iodine; the use of radioactive iodine; the administration of propylthiouracil, a drug which decreases the secretion of the thyroid hormone; and surgery.

(1) In administering Lugol's solution, with what should it be diluted to prevent burning?

(2) Two complications of a subtotal thyroidectomy are hemorrhage and paralysis of the vocal chords. Which anatomic structures near the thyroid gland contribute to the possibility of these complications?

(3) Another possible postoperative complication is thyroid crisis, which is an exaggeration of the symptoms of hyperthyroidism. Name the symptoms which may indicate the onset of the crisis.

(4) Following surgery, the danger of aspirating mouth secretions is great because the throat reflexes may be dull. In which position should the patient be placed to enable the secretions to drain from the mouth?

3. Diabetes mellitus is a condition in which there is an insufficient amount of insulin in the body. You will remember that carbohydrates in the diet are digested into simple sugars and converted into glycogen to be stored in the liver and used by the body cells. Insulin is necessary for this transformation of glucose into glycogen, both in the liver and in the tissues.

A. Discuss the incidence of diabetes mellitus.

B. Name the organizations which are interested in diabetes mellitus.

C. List the symptoms of the disease.

D. The glucose tolerance test is sometimes used in diagnosing the disease. Normally when one eats a large portion of sugar, the amount of sugar in the blood rises temporarily but will return to normal within 2 to 2-1/2 hours. In the glucose tolerance test, the patient is given a large amount of glucose, and tests are made at various intervals to determine the amount of sugar in the blood.

(1) How much sugar is normally present in the blood?

(2) Describe the steps of the glucose tolerance test.

(3) How is the patient prepared for the test?

E. Describe the fractional urinalysis.

F. Name a method used to test the urine of diabetics.

G. If diabetes mellitus is to be treated effectively, the patient must have some understanding of the disease. The treatment, in general, consists of the administration of insulin and the regulation of the diet. A mild diabetes may be controlled by diet alone.

(1) How is insulin measured?

(2) Where is commercial insulin obtained?

(3) Complete the table.

TYPE OF INSULIN	ONSET OF EFFECT	PEAK OF EFFECT	DURATION OF EFFECT
Regular			
Crystalline			
Protamine zinc			
Globin			
NPH			

(4) Which type of insulin is used in an emergency situation? Why?

(5) Where should insulin be stored?

(6) Name several factors which affect the diet prescribed for the patient.

(7) How may the type of insulin the patient is receiving affect the distribution of calories taken in a twenty-four hour period?

(8) What kinds of foods should the diabetic avoid?

(9) List the complications of diabetes.

(10) Name ten things which should be taught to the diabetic before his discharge from the hospital.

GENERAL NURSING CARE

Multiple Choice. Circle the number preceding the correct answer to each statement.

Mr. D., age thirty-five, was admitted to the hospital with a diagnosis of diabetic coma.

1. Diabetes mellitus is

a. More prevalent among the Jews.	1. All but c
b. Hereditary.	2. All but e
c. Caused by pregnancy.	3. a, b
d. More prevalent among the obese.	4. All but a
e. Curable.	5. a, b, d

2. Diabetes mellitus results from a disturbance of the

   1. Pituitary.
   2. Thyroid.
   3. Pancreas.
   4. Kidneys.
   5. Adrenals.

3. Diabetic coma is a condition caused by

a. The rapid metabolism of fat.	1. a, b
b. An accumulation of acetone bodies.	2. a, b, e
c. Too much insulin.	3. c, d
d. An insufficient amount of glucose in the blood	4. All
e. Hypotension.	5. None

4. Mr. D.'s symptoms were

a. Sweetish odor of the breath.	1. All but c
b. Profuse perspiration.	2. All but b
c. Flushed, dry skin.	3. b, e
d. Nausea and vomiting.	4. a, c, d
e. Trembling of the hands.	5. All

5. The emergency treatment for diabetic coma is

   1. The administration of sugar.
   2. The administration of orange juice.
   3. Insulin.
   4. Oxygen.
   5. None of these.

6. Some of the symptoms of diabetes mellitus are

a. Weight gain.
b. Polydipsia.
c. Excessive urination.
d. Glycosuria.
e. Increased hunger.

1. All
2. b, c, e
3. All but d
4. All but a
5. c, e

7. The duration of the action of protamine zinc insulin is

1. 24 hours or more.
2. 12 to 24 hours.
3. 8 to 10 hours.
4. 2 to 4 hours.

8. Mr. D. is to receive regular insulin a.c. The insulin should be given

1. Thirty minutes after meals.
2. Thirty minutes before meals.
3. One hour after meals.
4. One hour before meals.

9. The insulin is administered by holding the syringe at what angle to the skin?

1. 15 degrees.
2. 30 degrees.
3. 45 degrees.
4. 60 degrees.

10. Diabetics are prone to

a. Infections.
b. Gangrene.
c. Arteriosclerosis.
d. Hyperthyroidism.
e. Diabetes insipidus.

1. None
2. All
3. All but e
4. a, b
5. a, b, c

11. In teaching Mr. D. the care of the feet, the following facts should be stressed:

a. Shoes should fit tightly.
b. Hot foot soaks should be used at least once weekly.
c. Calluses should be removed only with a sterile razor blade.
d. Nails should be cut in a V shape.
e. Strong antiseptics should be used frequently to prevent gangrene.

1. All
2. None
3. All but d
4. b, e
5. All but a

12. In calculating the diet, the physician will take into consideration the patient's

a. Age.
b. Weight.
c. Sex.
d. Activity.
e. Severity of the disease.

1. All
2. All but d
3. a, b, c
4. All but a
5. e

13. In planning the diet, the nurse must remember that one gram of carbohydrates yields

1. 9 calories.
2. 8 calories.
3. 6 calories.
4. 4 calories.

14. A 3 per cent vegetable is

1. Carrots.
2. Broccoli.
3. Peas.
4. Lima beans.

15. When a diabetic patient refuses to eat all the food on his tray,

a. The doctor should be notified immediately.	1. a, b
b. Other foods which the patient likes will be substituted.	2. c
c. A gastrostomy feeding will be given.	3. a, c
d. A lump of sugar should be substituted.	4. a, d
	5. b

16. Diabetes insipidus results from a hypofunction of the

1. Pancreas.
2. Pituitary.
3. Adrenal.
4. Gonads.

17. The basal metabolism rate

a. Measures the rate at which the body uses oxygen.	1. a
b. Is elevated in hyperthyroidism.	2. a, c
c. Is recorded as numbers in plus or minus zero.	3. All but c
d. Is based on age, weight, height and sex.	4. All
e. Measures the metabolism rate when the patient is at rest.	5. None

18. The common complications of thyroid surgery are

a. Pneumonia.	1. All
b. Embolus.	2. None
c. Thyroid crisis.	3. All but b
d. Vocal chord paralysis.	4. All but a
e. Hemorrhage.	5. c, d, e

19. A symptom of all of the postoperative complications of the thyroidectomy is

1. Difficulty in breathing.
2. Hematemesis.
3. Edema.
4. Flushed skin.

20. Lugol's solution is a drug preparation of

    1. Thyroxin.
    2. Sodium chloride.
    3. Iodine.
    4. Radioisotopes.

Medication Review. Match Column I with Column II

Column I	Column II
a. Oral diabetic drug	______ 1. Tapazole
b. Checks secretion of thyroid hormone	______ 2. Crystalline insulin
c. Stimulates adrenal to secrete cortisone	______ 3. Orinase
d. Action time same as regular insulin	______ 4. ACTH
e. Supplements thyroid deficiency	______ 5. Diabinese
f. Insulin with a long-lasting effect	______ 6. Parathyroid extract
g. Regulates use of calcium in body	______ 7. Thyroid extract
h. Iodine preparation	______ 8. Propylthiouracil
	______ 9. Protamine zinc
	______ 10. Lugol's solution

Chapter 40

DISEASES OF THE NERVOUS SYSTEM

ANATOMY AND PHYSIOLOGY REVIEW
DIAGNOSTIC PROCEDURES
DISEASE CONDITIONS: CEREBRAL VASCULAR ACCIDENT, EPILEPSY, ANTERIOR POLIOMYELITIS, MULTIPLE SCLEROSIS, SKULL INJURIES, SPINAL COLUMN INJURIES
GENERAL NURSING CARE

REFERENCES

Culver, V.: Modern Bedside Nursing, Chapters 15 and 48.
Hoffman, C. P., Lipkin, G. P., and Thompson, E. M.: Simplified Nursing, Chapter 38.
Johnston, D. F.: Total Patient Care, Chapter 17.
Keane, C. B.: Essentials of Nursing, Chapter 17.
Mason, M. A.: Basic Medical and Surgical Nursing, Chapter 21.
Rapier, D. K., et al.: Practical Nursing, pp. 427-432.
Thompson, E., and Murphy, C.: Textbook of Basic Nursing, Chapter 43.

JOURNALS

Cooper, Irving S.: Cryogenic neurosurgery. J. Practical Nursing, 18:21, Sept. 1968.
Magee, Kenneth R.: Myasthenia gravis. J. Practical Nursing, 15:23, Nov. 1965.
Simmons, James Q.: Nursing the multiple sclerosis patient. J. Practical Nursing, 18:22, Nov. 1968.
Slosberg, Paul S.: Hypotension: treatment of intracranial aneurysm. J. Practical Nursing, 15:27, Oct. 1965.
White, Paul Dudley: Strokes: prevention, diagnosis and patient care. J. Practical Nursing, 15:24, Oct. 1965.

ANATOMY AND PHYSIOLOGY REVIEW

True or False. Circle T if the statement is true; F if the statement is false. Correct the statements that are false by crossing out the incorrect word or words and writing the correct word or words in the space above.

T F 1. The cerebrum is the largest part of the brain.

T F 2. In the spinal cord, the gray matter is on the outside and the white matter is on the inside.

T F 3. The covering of the brain and spinal cord is called the neuron.

T F 4. The nervous system functions on the basis of sensory and motor reflexes.

T F 5. The nerve cell is called myelin sheath.

DIAGNOSTIC PROCEDURES

Complete the table.

DIAGNOSTIC TEST	PREPARATION OF PATIENT
Lumbar puncture	
Encephalogram	

COMMON DISEASE CONDITIONS

1. Cerebral vascular accident, also called apoplexy and stroke, is a condition in which the blood vessels of the brain are affected by a rupture causing hemorrhage, thrombosis or embolism. Hypertension is a predisposing factor to cerebral accident. In a cerebral hemorrhage, the blood which escapes from the ruptured blood vessel accumulates and causes pressure on the surrounding brain tissue. The symptoms depend on the location and extent of the bleeding. When either a cerebral thrombosis or embolism occurs, a portion of the brain tissue is damaged because the blood supply to the part is blocked off.

A. Define:

(1) Hemiplegia

(2) Coma

(3) Convulsion

(4) Aphasia

B. What are the symptoms of a cerebral accident?

C. Discuss the reasons why each of the following is important in the nursing care of the patient.

(1) Expert skin care

(2) Special mouth care

(3) Occasional use of bed sides

(4) Attention to good body alignment

(5) An encouraging attitude on the part of the nurse

D. List five exercises which the nurse may encourage the patient to do while confined to bed.

2. Epilepsy is a condition in which the patient has a tendency toward periodic episodes of loss of consciousness, frequently accompanied by convulsions. The exact cause of epilepsy is unknown. The tendency toward the disease seems to be hereditary.

A. In what age group does the disease usually manifest itself?

B. Define each type of seizure:

(1) Jacksonian

(2) Grand mal

(3) Petit mal

C. What specific points should the nurse observe and record concerning a seizure?

D. What is the action of each drug used in the treatment?

(1) Phenobarbital

(2) Dilantin sodium

(3) Tridione

(4) Mesantoin

3. Anterior poliomyelitis, or infantile paralysis, is an infectious disease caused by a virus. The inflammation occurs in the anterior portion of the spinal cord. It will be remembered from the study of anatomy that this is the portion of the spinal cord which contains the motor reflex nerves.

A. Prevention:

B. Symptoms:

C. Treatment:

4. Multiple sclerosis is a disease which, for some unknown reason, destroys the myelin sheath of the nerves. The myelin sheath covers the entire length of the nerve fiber and acts something like insulation on an electric wire. When the insulation is lacking, the nerve impulses are altered or may be stopped completely.

A. Symptoms:

B. Age group most commonly affected:

C. Treatment:

D. What is the name and address of the national organization which is doing research in this field?

5. Skull injuries may result in injury to the brain. The injury may result from a blow which causes a hemorrhage between the skull and the dura (extradural hemorrhage) or between the dura and the brain (subdural hemorrhage). The slow bleeding forms a hematoma which increases in size and causes pressure on the brain. In skull fractures a portion of the broken bone may be pressed against the brain and cause pressure symptoms, or the fractured bone may cause unrepairable damage to the brain tissue.

A. Define cerebral concussion.

B. What are the symptoms of brain injury?

C. What is the first-aid treatment for a head injury?

6. Spinal column injuries are dangerous because of the possibility of damage to the spinal cord. The spinal cord is a soft structure like the brain and does not withstand minor trauma or bacterial invasion. When the spinal cord is injured in the cervical area, a paralysis of the four extremities and the muscles of the chest and abdomen occurs. The prognosis for this type of injury is poor. A lumbar and thoracic injury may result in a paralysis of both legs and loss of bladder control. The first-aid treatment for one suspected of having a fracture or dislocation of the spinal column is very important. The patient should not be moved until medical help is available.

A. Define:

(1) Paraplegia

(2) Quadraplegia

B. The posture of the patient with a spinal column injury is important in order to treat the condition and to prevent further damage. The Foster bed is frequently used to keep the patient in the proper position.

(1) Describe the Foster bed.

(2) Describe the methods used to turn a patient with this condition who is not in a Foster bed.

C. Why must special emphasis be placed on

(1) Skin care?

(2) Rehabilitation?

7. Other conditions: Use each of the terms in a sentence showing that you understand the meaning.

A. Neuralgia

B. Neuritis

C. Meningitis

D. Encephalitis

E. Herpes zoster

F. Cerebral palsy

GENERAL NURSING CARE

True or False. Circle T if the statement is true; F if the statement if false.

T F 1. The tendency toward epilepsy may be inherited.
T F 2. Most epileptics are mentally deficient.
T F 3. There are several good drugs on the market which cure epilepsy.
T F 4. Most patients suffering from diseases of the nervous system require a great deal of efficient around-the-clock nursing care.
T F 5. All cases of poliomyelitis leave the patient crippled.
T F 6. Passive exercise is exercise which the patient can do himself.
T F 7. Multiple sclerosis is caused by a filtrable virus.
T F 8. Encephalitis is sometimes called apoplexy.
T F 9. Isolation technique is used in the care of the patient with meningitis.
T F 10. The patient who appears to be in a semicomatose state cannot hear.

Match each condition with the correct first-aid treatment.

Condition	Treatment
a. Cerebral accident	_____ 1. Keep the patient flat; do not move
b. Epileptic seizure	_____ 2. Put the patient to bed
c. Possible skull injury	_____ 3. Closely observe the reflexes for at least twenty-four hours
d. Spinal cord injury	_____ 4. Do not restrain

Multiple Choice. Circle the number preceding the correct answer to each statement.

Practical Nurse S. is going to stay with Mary, a ten-year-old epileptic, for several days while Mary's mother is away on a business trip.

1. Before Mary's mother leaves, Practical Nurse S. will inquire about the following:

a. The frequency of the seizures	1. All
b. The type of seizures	2. None
c. The time of day the seizure usually occurs	3. a
d. The type of medication given	4. a, c, e
e. The conditions which contribute to the occurrence of the seizure	5. All but b

2. Mary usually knows when a seizure will begin. The warning before a seizure is called

   1. Frothing.
   2. Aura.
   3. Jacksonian.
   4. Tonic stage.

3. During a seizure Mary becomes rigid and cyanotic, and the muscles of the entire body alternately contract and relax. This type of seizure is

   1. Grand mal.
   2. Petit mal.
   3. Jacksonian.

4. During the seizure, a padded tongue blade should be placed between the teeth to prevent

   1. Suffocation.
   2. Injury to the tongue.
   3. Dyspnea.
   4. Frothing at the mouth.

5. Following the seizure, the nurse will arrange for Mary to

   1. Watch television.
   2. Play.
   3. Eat.
   4. Rest.

Mrs. M., age sixty, had a cerebral vascular accident and was admitted to the hospital in a coma.

6. Coma means that Mrs. M.

a. Has an elevated temperature.	1. All
b. Is delirious.	2. None
c. Has hallucinations.	3. All but a
d. Does not respond to external stimuli.	4. b, d
e. Has lost awareness of her surroundings.	5. d, e

7. A left-sided hemiplegia resulted. The side of the brain which was affected was the

   1. Left side.
   2. Right side.

8. The nurse observed that the patient had a speech difficulty. The term for this is

   1. Quadriplegia.
   2. Paralysis.
   3. Aphasia.
   4. Delirium.

9. Nursing care for the patient includes

a. A system for communicating.	1. All but d
b. Special mouth care.	2. a, c, e
c. Expert skin care.	3. a, b, c
d. Eye care.	4. All but e
e. Changing the position frequently.	5. All

10. The management of the paralysis includes

a. The use of a footboard.
b. Keeping the hand open.
c. Using support to keep the leg from rolling outward.
d. Keeping the foot of the bed elevated.
e. Allowing the patient to lie only on her back or abdomen.

1. All
2. All but e
3. a
4. a, b, c
5. None

11. A decubitus ulcer can be prevented by

a. Frequent alcohol rubs.
b. Daily bathing.
c. Frequent change in position.
d. Keeping the sheets smooth.
e. Exercise.

1. All but e
2. a, b, c
3. All but b
4. a
5. All

12. In giving an enema to Mrs. M., the nurse will need

1. Less solution than usual.
2. More solution than usual.
3. Extra protection for the bed.
4. An additional supply of lubricant.

13. The recovery of such a patient

a. Is hopeless in the majority of cases.
b. Is slow.
c. Depends on the severity of brain damage.
d. Depends somewhat on the patient's mental attitude.
e. Can be complete only for those patients who have not been in a coma.

1. b, c, d
2. c
3. c, e
4. All
5. None

14. The Kenney treatment for poliomyelitis consists of

a. Immobilizing the affected part.
b. Exercise.
c. Massage.
d. The application of hot moist packs.
e. The use of splints.

1. All
2. All but e
3. b, c, d
4. d
5. c

15. The Foster bed is built for the purpose of allowing the patient to lie on

1. His back only.
2. His back and abdomen.
3. His abdomen only.
4. Both sides, back and abdomen.

Medication Review. Match each medication with its action.

Action	Medication
a. Stimulant	______ 1. Morphine
b. Depressant	______ 2. Caffeine
c. Opiate	______ 3. Alcohol
d. Hypnotic	______ 4. Chloral hydrate
e. Tranquilizer	______ 5. Codeine
f. Barbiturate	______ 6. Benzedrine
	______ 7. Novocain
	______ 8. Thorazine
	______ 9. Nembutal
	______ 10. Dexedrine

Chapter 41

DISEASES OF THE SPECIAL SENSES

ANATOMY AND PHYSIOLOGY REVIEW
DIAGNOSTIC TESTS
DISEASE CONDITIONS: DEAFNESS, INFECTIONS, FOREIGN BODIES, GLAUCOMA, CATARACT, ERRORS OF REFRACTION
GENERAL NURSING CARE

REFERENCES

Culver, V.: Modern Bedside Nursing, Chapters 16 and 49.
Hoffman, C. P., Lipkin, G. P., and Thompson, E. M.: Simplified Nursing, Chapter 39.
Johnston, D. F.: Total Patient Care, Chapter 18.
Keane, C. B.: Essentials of Nursing, Chapter 19.
Mason, M. A.: Basic Medical and Surgical Nursing, Chapters 22-23.
Thompson, E., and Murphy, C.: Textbook of Basic Nursing, Chapter 45.

JOURNAL

Fogel, Howard H.: The patient with a hearing aid. Bedside Nurse, 1:19, July-Aug. 1968.

The Ear

ANATOMY AND PHYSIOLOGY REVIEW

1. Label the parts of the ear in Figure 52.

   A. Pinna ; earlobe

   B. Auditory canal

   C. Malleus

   D. Anvil

   E. Stirrup

   F. Cochlea

   G. Tympanic membrane

   H. Eustachian tube

2. What are the two functions of the ear?

3. Complete.

   A. The external auditory canal is about __________ inches long.

   B. The middle ear opens into the ______________________, a small canal about _________ inches long, which leads into the throat.

   C. The _________________ ear picks up sound waves and sends the impulses to the brain by means of a spiral coil containing ___________________________.

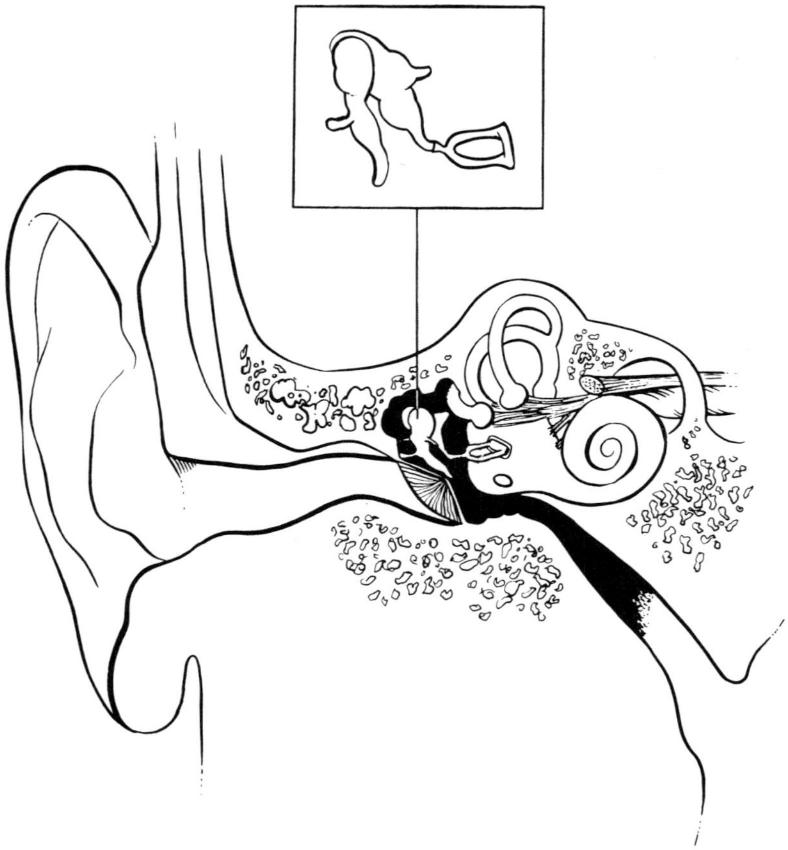

Fig. 51. The human ear. (McKean, I.: Anatomy and Physiology Laboratory Manual and Study Guide.)

DIAGNOSTIC TESTS

1. Explain how each is used in diagnosing diseases of the ear.

   A. Tuning fork

   B. Otoscope

   C. Audiometer

DISEASE CONDITIONS

1. Deafness is the loss or impairment of hearing.

   A. Outline the route of sound waves from the time they enter the auditory canal to the time they are picked up by the auditory nerve.

   B. What abnormalities may interfere with the conduction of the sound waves?

   C. Which of these abnormalities may be only temporary?

   D. What special considerations should the nurse make in caring for a patient who is

      (1) Partially deaf?

      (2) Totally deaf?

2. Ear infections include otomycosis, a fungus infection of the external ear; otitis media, an infection of the middle ear; and labyrinthitis, inflammation of the semicircular canals.

   A. Discuss the prevention of ear infections.

   B. What is a possible complication of otitis media?

   C. What is the treatment for

      (1) Otomycosis?

      (2) Otitis media?

      (3) Labyrinthitis?

   D. Describe the action of each drug

      (1) Penicillin

      (2) Demerol hydrochloride

(3). Sulfa drugs

(4) Seconal

(5) Hydrogen peroxide

3. Foreign bodies in the external ear should always be removed by a physician. The method of removal depends on the type of object lodged in the ear.

A. Why are vegetables such as a dried pea or bean removed with the use of a dehydrating agent (ether) rather than water?

B. What danger lies in having an unskilled person attempt to remove a foreign body from the ear?

The Eye

ANATOMY AND PHYSIOLOGY REVIEW

1. Color the parts of the eye in Figure 53.

   A. Retina - yellow
   B. Sclera - red
   C. Choroid - blue
   D. Aqueous humor - green

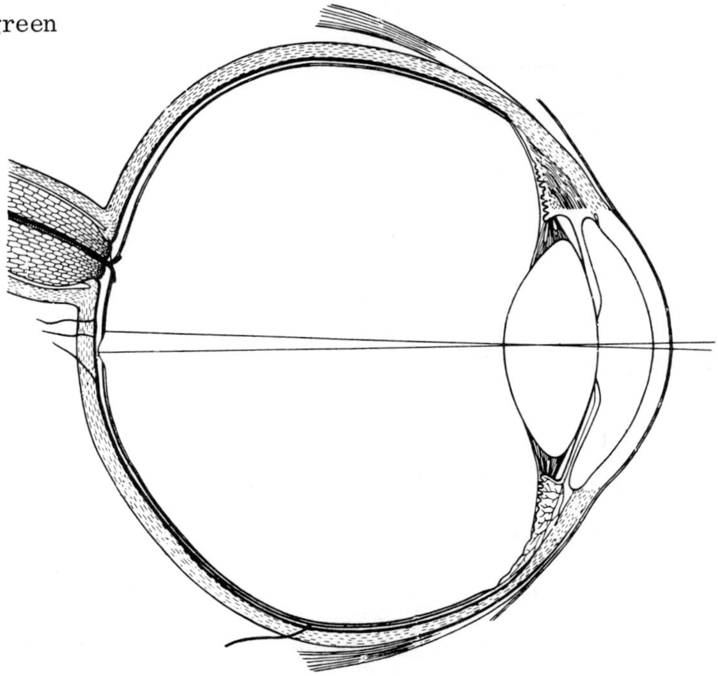

Fig. 52. The human eye. (Courtesy, General Biological Supply House, Inc., Chicago, Illinois.)

2. Label the parts of the eye.

   A. Iris
   B. Ciliary muscle
   C. Pupil
   D. Vitreous humor
   E. Cornea
   F. Optic nerve
   G. Lens

3. Complete.

   A. The eye is located in the ______________ and is surrounded by ______________ tissue.

   B. Light enters the eye through the ________________.

C. The _______ in the center of the iris, regulates the amount of light entering the eye by ______________________________ .

D. The ______________, located behind the iris, helps to focus the light rays on the ____________________, the part of the eye which receives the light image and sends it to the optic nerve.

E. The _____________, _______________ and ______________ are accessory organs to the eye.

4. Project. Make an eye safety poster on a sheet of paper 8-1/2 x 11 inches in size.

DIAGNOSTIC TESTS

1. What abnormalities may be discovered with the use of

A. Ophthalmoscope?

B. Snellen charts?

2. Here are some words you should know. Make a complete sentence using each.

A. Refraction

B. Accommodation

C. Optometrist

D. Optician

E. Photophobia

DISEASE CONDITIONS

1. Eye infections include conjunctivitis, inflammation of the conjunctiva; keratitis, inflammation of the cornea; retinitis, inflammation of the retina; and iritis, inflammation of the iris. Conjunctivitis and keratitis may be caused by gonorrhea.

A. Which of these infections enters the eye from

(1) The outside?

(2) The blood stream?

B. Which infection is commonly called pink eye?

C. Which procedure in the immediate care of the newborn is performed to prevent gonorrhea of the newborn?

D. Discuss the proper hygiene of the eyes and its importance in the prevention of eye inflammations.

2. Glaucoma is a condition resulting from inadequate drainage of the fluid from within the eyeball. The impairment in the drainage process causes an excessive amount of fluid to collect within the eyeball. This results in increased pressure and eventually will result in hardening of the fluid and blindness.

A. Cause:

B. Symptoms:

C. Treatment:

3. A cataract is a condition in which the lens is cloudy. The only effective treatment for this condition is the surgical removal of the lens.

A. Cause:

B. Symptoms:

4. Errors of refraction.

A. Define and give the lay term for

(1) Myopia

(2) Hyperopia

(3) Astigmatism

B. Discuss the treatment of each of the above.

5. A common source of injury to the eye is foreign bodies.

A. What is the first-aid treatment for the removal of foreign bodies from the eye?

B. What dangers lie in the removal of foreign bodies?

6. An aspect of treatment related to the eye which may be of interest to the student practical nurse is the corneal transplantation. What information can you find concerning this?

GENERAL NURSING CARE FOR THE EAR AND THE EYE

1. True or False. Circle T if the statement is true; F if the statement is false. Correct the statements that are false by crossing out the incorrect word or words and writing the correct word or words above.

T F 1. Eyes that are being unbandaged for the first time postoperatively should be protected from the light by having the room moderately darkened.

T F 2. When instilling eyedrops, pull the lower lid downward, request the patient to look downward, and allow the drops to fall in the outer aspect of the eye.

T F 3. In administering eyedrops, one should be careful not to touch the eyeball with the dropper.

T F 4. When applying ointment to the eye, place the prescribed ointment under the inner portion of the upper lid and instruct the patient to hold the eye open for several minutes.

T F 5. When instilling drops in the ear, pull the ear lobe upward and backward on the adult, and downward and backward on the child.

T F 6. Before an eye or ear irrigation is performed, the temperature of the solution should be tested with a bath thermometer.

T F 7. The application of a small coat of petroleum to the eyelid before applying hot moist compresses aids in relieving pain and congestion.

T F 8. Ear irrigations should be given under low pressure to prevent damage to the auditory nerve.

T F 9. The abbreviation O.D. means right eye; O.S. means left eye.

T F 10. If both eyes or both ears are to be irrigated, separate sets of equipment will be needed.

T F 11. The hospital stay for patients with eye surgery has been decreased.

T F 12. Symptoms of atropine toxicity are nausea, vomiting and severe rash.

T F 13. It is essential in feeding the patient who cannot see to have him eat as rapidly as possible in order to eliminate the embarrassment he experiences from the procedure.

T F 14. A patient who intends to purchase a hearing aid should first consult the nurse in order to know which type will be of most benefit.

T F 15. During hospitalization, the responsibility for the care of the prosthetic eye is assumed totally by the patient.

2. Discussion.

A. List five special considerations the nurse should make in the care of the blind patient.

B. In your community where can Talking Book records be obtained?

C. Recent advances in eye surgery have brought about changes in the postoperative care of the patient. What is the postoperative care of the cataract patient in your hospital?

3. Medication Review. Match the medication with its action.

Action	Medication
a. Dilates pupil	____ 1. Pilocarpine
b. Antiseptic	____ 2. Penicillin
c. Constricts pupil	____ 3. Silver nitrate
d. Antibiotic	____ 4. Atropine
e. Cleansing agent	____ 5. Normal saline

Chapter 42

DISEASES OF THE SKIN

ANATOMY AND PHYSIOLOGY REVIEW
DISEASE CONDITIONS: ACNE VULGARIS, ATHLETE'S FOOT, RINGWORM, IMPETIGO CONTAGIOSA, ECZEMA, PSORIASIS
GENERAL NURSING CARE

REFERENCES

Culver, V.: Modern Bedside Nursing, Chapter 49.
Hoffman, C. P., Lipkin, G. P., and Thompson, E. M.: Simplified Nursing, Chapter 30.
Johnston, D. F.: Total Patient Care, Chapter 19.
Keane, C. B.: Essentials of Nursing, Chapter 10.
Mason, M. A.: Basic Medical and Surgical Nursing, Chapter 34.
Thompson, E., and Murphy, C.: Textbook of Basic Nursing, Chapter 34.

ANATOMY AND PHYSIOLOGY REVIEW

1. Color the parts of the skin shown in Figure 54.

   A. Sebaceous gland and duct - red
   B. Hair root - blue
   C. Sweat gland - green
   D. Arrector muscle - brown
   E. Epidermis - yellow

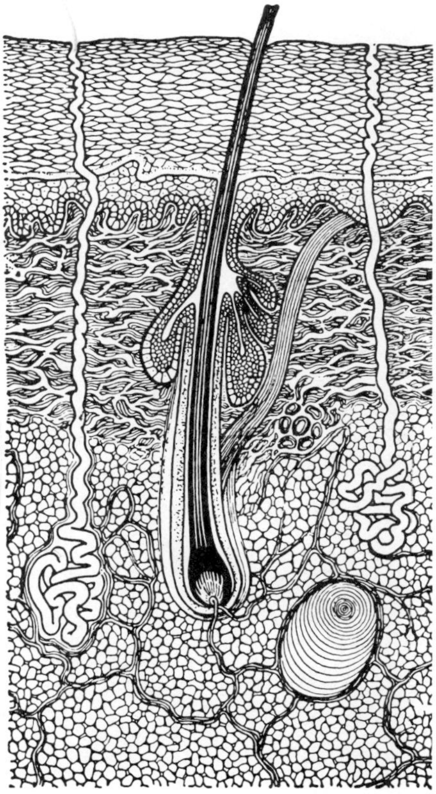

Fig. 53. The Skin. Modified from Tuttle and Schottelius, and Anthony, C. P.: Structure and Function of the Body 3rd ed. St. Louis, The C. V. Mosby Co., 1968

2. What are the functions of the skin? Protection. sensory organ - to regulate the body temperature

3. Discuss the care of

   A. Dry skin

   B. Oily skin

4. What changes in the skin occur with age?

DISEASE CONDITIONS

1. Define:

   A. Macule : a discolored circumscribed area not causing skin elevation

   B. Wheal

   C. Papule ; a circumscribed area causing skin elevation

   D. Pustule ; a papule filled with pus

   E. Vesicle ; a papule filled with clear fluid

2. Match each term with the definition.

Term		Definition
a. Dermatitis	d	1. Itching
b. Gangrene	c	2. Hives
c. Urticaria	b	3. Death of a tissue
d. Pruritus	a	4. Inflammation of the skin
e. Carbuncle	e	5. Deep-seated abscess

3. Complete the table.

CONDITION	CAUSE	SYMPTOMS	TREATMENT
Acne vulgaris			
Athlete's foot			
Ringworm			
Impetigo contagiosa			
Eczema			
Psoriasis			

GENERAL NURSING CARE

Multiple Choice. Circle the letter preceding the correct answer to each statement.

1. Vitamin A is sometimes increased in the diet to treat acne. The foods highest in vitamin A content are

   A. Fish liver oils and butter.
   B. Peas and lima beans.
   C. Strawberries and grapes.

2. Poison ivy is a form of

   A. Contact dermatitis.
   B. Eczema.
   C. Acne.

Miss K. visited her family physician because of the appearance of hives over her entire body.

3. The hives could be described as

   A. Pustules.
   B. Wheals.
   C. Nodules.

4. The physician believed that the condition was caused by an allergy to certain types of food. An allergy is

   A. A hyposensitivity to substances.
   B. Hypersensitivity to certain substances.
   C. Always manifested by itching.

5. In order to determine the cause of the allergy, the physician administered a sensitivity test. This was done by giving a small amount of solution intradermally. To give the injection, the physician would hold the syringe at what angle to the skin?

   A. 15 degrees.
   B. 45 degrees.
   C. 90 degrees.

6. Daily cornstarch baths were ordered. The office nurse instructed Miss K. in the procedure for taking the baths as follows:

   A. "Fill the tub half full of water, as warm as can be tolerated, and add two cups of starch to the water, stirring constantly. Remain in the tub twenty minutes. Dry vigorously with a bath towel."
   B. "Dissolve two cups of starch in cold water and add boiling water to form a paste. Add this mixture to a tub half full of tepid water. Remain in the tub about twenty minutes. To dry, do not rub, but pat gently with a towel."

C. "Dissolve one-half cup of starch in cold water and add boiling water to form a paste. Add this mixture to a tub half full of lukewarm water. Remain in the tub about one hour. To dry, do not rub, but pat gently with a towel."

Baby Jane, age six months, was admitted to the pediatric department with eczema.

7. Her rash was

   A. Dry and scaly.
   B. Moist and oozing.
   C. Either condition is possible.

8. The daily nursing care for Baby Jane included

   A. Soap and water baths.
   B. Methods employed to allay itching.
   C. The use of flannel instead of cotton knit bedclothes.
   D. All of these.

9. In order to prevent scratching, Baby Jane can be restrained sufficiently and yet retain a certain amount of freedom by

   A. Tying her arms loosely to the crib side.
   B. Placing rolls of cardboard over the arms to prevent bending of the elbows.
   C. Pinning the shirt sleeves to the bottom sheet.

10. An ointment was ordered. In applying the ointment, the nurse must always remember to

   A. Rub the ointment briskly on the skin with tongue blades and cover the area with gauze.
   B. Apply a thick coat of ointment.
   C. Remove thoroughly all the old ointment left on the skin before applying the new ointment.

Medication Review. Match Column I with Column II

Column I		Column II
a. A nonirritant used to remove ointment	e	1. Aluminum paste
b. Antihistamine	d	2. Calamine lotion
c. Systemic antifungal	a	3. Liquid petrolatum
d. An astringent and antipruritic	c	4. Griseofulvin
e. Used to protect skin from draining wounds	b	5. Pyribenzamine

Chapter 43

DISEASES OF THE REPRODUCTIVE SYSTEM

ANATOMY AND PHYSIOLOGY REVIEW
DIAGNOSTIC EXAMINATIONS
DISEASE CONDITIONS: INFLAMMATIONS, CYSTOCELE AND RECTOCELE, CYSTS AND TUMORS, UTERINE DISPLACEMENTS, ORCHITIS, BENIGN PROSTATIC HYPERTROPHY
GENERAL NURSING CARE

REFERENCES

Culver, V.: Modern Bedside Nursing, Chapters 13 and 47.
Hoffman, C. P., Lipkin, G. P., and Thompson, E. M.: Simplified Nursing, Chapter 36.
Johnston, D. F.: Total Patient Care, Chapter 15.
Keane, C. B.: Essentials of Nursing, Chapter 17.
Mason, M. A.: Basic Medical and Surgical Nursing, Chapter 20.
Rapier, D. K., et al.: Practical Nursing, pp. 425-427.
Thompson, E., and Murphy, C.: Textbook of Basic Nursing, pp. 530-537.

ANATOMY AND PHYSIOLOGY REVIEW

1. Name the functions of the parts of the female reproductive system.

   A. Ovaries

   B. Uterus

   C. Fallopian tubes

2. Color the parts of the female external genitalia shown in Figure 55.

   A. Clitoris - green
   B. Labia majora - blue
   C. Labia minora - red

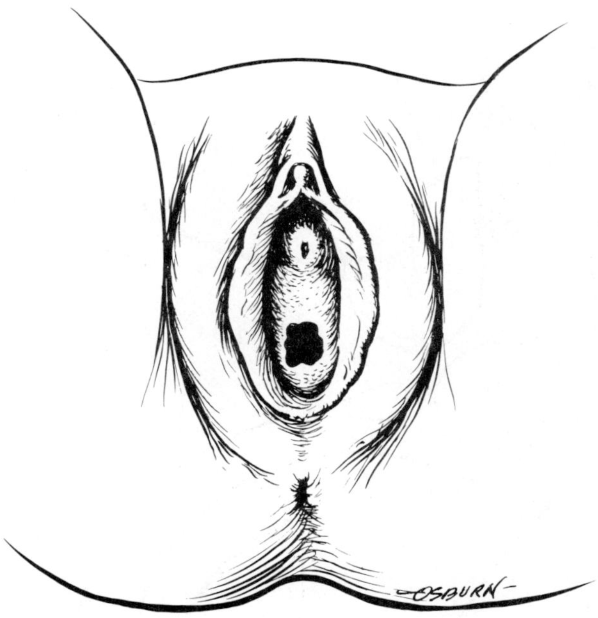

Fig. 54. Female external genitalia.

3. Label the parts of the female genitalia.

   A. Urethra
   B. Vagina
   C. Perineum
   D. Anus

4. Label the parts of the male reproductive system in Figure 55.

   A. Testes

   B. Prostate gland

   C. Scrotum

   D. Epididymis

   E. Seminal duct

   F. Seminal vesicle

   G. Urethra

   H. Penis

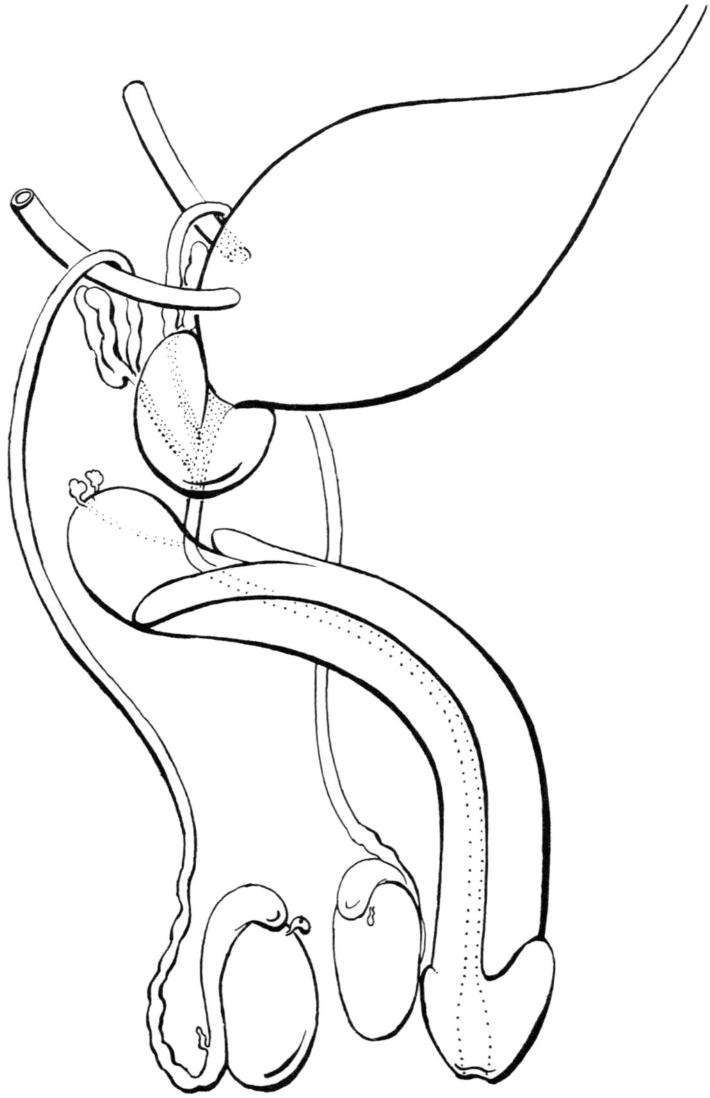

Fig. 55. Male reproductive organs. (Denoyer-Geppert Company, Chicago, Illinois.)

DIAGNOSTIC EXAMINATIONS

1. Complete the table.

EXAMINATION	DEFINITION	PREPARATION OF PATIENT
Rubin's test		
Papanicolaou smear		
Biopsy		

DISEASE CONDITIONS

1. Match each gynecological term with the correct definition.

Term		Definition
a. Amenorrhea	_____	1. Inability to conceive
b. Menstruation	_____	2. Surgical removal of the breast
c. Dysmenorrhea	_____	3. Surgical removal of the uterus
d. Hysterectomy	_____	4. Absence of menstruation
e. Metrorrhagia	_____	5. Uterine lining
f. Menopause	_____	6. Menses
g. Leukorrhea	_____	7. Painful menstruation
h. Sterility	_____	8. A thick, white vaginal discharge
i. Mastectomy	_____	9. The period when menstruation ceases
j. Endometrium	_____	10. Bleeding between menstrual periods

2. Inflammations of the female reproductive system. Complete the table.

INFLAMMATION	CAUSE	SYMPTOMS	TREATMENT
Vulvitis			
Vaginitis			
Salpingitis			
Gonorrhea			

3. A cystocele is a herniation or prolapse of the bladder caused by a tear or weakening of the fascia surrounding the cervix. A rectocele is a herniation of the rectum toward the vagina caused by a laceration or weakening of the posterior vaginal fascia.

A. List the symptoms of each condition.

B. What are the terms for the surgical repair of each condition?

4. The common cysts and benign tumors of the female reproductive system include fibroid tumor of the uterus, ovarian cyst, cervical polyp, and benign tumors of the breast. The treatment for these is surgery. Carcinoma may occur in any of the glands of the female reproductive system.

A. Arrange and number the parts of the female reproductive system according to the incidence of cancer of the part. Begin with the organ most frequently affected.

B. How does cancer of the reproductive system rank among the incidence of cancer in other parts of the female body?

C. List five ways in which the practical nurse can aid in the early detection of cancer.

5. Uterine displacements include prolapse, anteflexion and retroversion. Define each.

Anteflexion and retroversion very seldom cause discomfort and, therefore, need no treatment. If a prolapse of the uterus is mild or partial, it is treated by a repair of the pelvic floor. If the prolapse is severe or complete, it is treated by a vaginal hysterectomy. The usual complaint of a woman with a prolapsed uterus is that when she is standing, it feels as if her "insides were falling out."

6. Orchitis is inflammation of the testis, which may be a complication of gonorrhea or the mumps. A bilateral orchitis may cause sterility.

A. Symptoms:

B. Treatment:

7. Benign prostatic hypertrophy, or enlargement of the prostate, is a common condition which occurs in over one-third of all males over fifty years of age. The exact cause of this condition is unknown, but it is believed that it is due to an endocrine disturbance. Because of the location of the prostate, the symptoms are disturbances of urination.

A. Symptoms:

B. What is tidal drainage?

C. What methods are used to control hemorrhage postoperatively?

D. What procedure is performed postoperatively to prevent the indwelling catheter from becoming clogged with blood clots?

E. What is the incidence of cancer of the prostate among this age group?

GENERAL NURSING CARE

1. Place a red line under each article which the nurse should assemble in preparation for a routine vaginal examination.

A. Catheter
B. Light
C. Lubricant
D. Urine specimen bottle
E. Cotton applicators
F. Gauze squares
G. Kelly clamp (long)
H. Vaginal speculum
I. Emesis basin
J. Douche nozzle

2. Which parts of the body does the physician examine in a routine vaginal examination?

3. Multiple Choice. Circle the number preceding the correct answer to each statement.

Mrs. B., age sixty, completed her menopause several years ago. She seems to be in perfect health but has an occasional bloody vaginal discharge.

(1) This occasional bleeding

(a) Is normal following menopause, providing the bleeding is not profuse.
(b) May indicate the presence of carcinoma.
(c) Is called leukorrhea.

(2) Mrs. B. decided to visit a clinic even though she felt fine. In preparation for a vaginal examination, the nurse placed the patient in the correct position, which was

(a) Trendelenburg.
(b) Lithotomy.
(c) Fowler's.

(3) Mrs. B. was naturally a little tense. To make the patient feel at ease while preparing her for the vaginal examination, the nurse should

(a) Work rapidly.
(b) Satisfactorily explain each step of the preparation.
(c) Leave the examining room for a few minutes.

(4) The nurse can help the patient relax during a vaginal examination by

(a) Holding her hand.
(b) Carrying on a continual conversation to divert the patient's mind.
(c) Asking the patient to breathe deeply through her mouth.

(5) The physician decided to take a Papanicolaou smear. For this the doctor will need a special wooden spatula and

(a) Sterile test tubes.
(b) Microscopic slides.
(c) Three sterile basins.

(6) The gynecological nurse must be an especially good teacher because

(a) Most women prefer to discuss their gynecological problems with someone of their own sex.
(b) The female reproductive system requires more hygienic care than any other bodily system.
(c) Most doctors feel that this is a nursing responsibility.

Mrs. S. was admitted to the hospital with a severely prolapsed uterus and was to have a vaginal hysterectomy. Her preoperative preparation included a vaginal irrigation of potassium permanganate 1:8000.

(7) This procedure was done to

(a) Treat the pelvic inflammation.
(b) Relieve pain.
(c) Cleanse the vaginal canal.

(8) In order to insure proper results in giving the douche, the nurse should

(a) Slowly rotate the douche nozzle.
(b) Hold the irrigating can 24 inches above the pelvis.
(c) Place the patient in Sim's position.

(9) In shaving Mrs. S. in preparation for surgery, the site to be prepared includes

(a) The pubic, perineal and rectal areas and the inner thighs.
(b) The entire body from the waist on down to the knees, both front and back.
(c) The pubic hair.

(10) Inserting a catheter was another preoperative order. When cleansing the labia, before inserting the catheter, the nurse cleanses

(a) The labia majora, then the labia minora and the urinary meatus, using one cotton ball once and wiping downward each time.
(b) The entire perineum, using three to four cotton balls for each cleansing stroke.
(c) The urinary meatus, using one cotton ball with each stroke.

(11) The following would be considered a break in the sterile technique used in catheterizing Mrs. S.:

(a) Opening the outer wrapper of the tray before putting on the gloves.
(b) Separating the labia with the left hand; cleansing the area with cotton balls and forceps held in the right hand.
(c) Removing the left hand from the labia and inserting the catheter.

Mrs. M. has just returned from the recovery room following a vaginal plastic operation.

(12) A nursing measure which will probably be carried out to help prevent contamination of the perineal sutures is

(a) The application of hot moist compresses.
(b) An external irrigation of the perineal area following each voiding and defecation.
(c) The use of the heat lamp.

(13) Until the suture line was healed, Mrs. M. was on a low residue diet to help keep the bowels inactive, thus preventing strain on the operative site. The food lowest in residue is

(a) Sliced chicken.
(b) Peas.
(c) Sliced fresh peaches.

Mrs. K. had a left radical mastectomy performed for the removal of a malignant tumor.

(14) An aspect of the treatment which may cause emotional tension is the fear of

(a) Disfigurement and rejection.
(b) The loss of the use of her left arm.
(c) Pain.

(15) The surgeon prescribed arm exercises to begin 24 hours after surgery. These are done to

(a) Prevent pain.
(b) Prevent loss of arm function.
(c) Prevent metastasis.

(16) In cases of sterility among marriage partners, the percentage of infertility among the males is

(a) 30 to 35 per cent.
(b) 50 to 60 per cent.
(c) 70 to 75 per cent.

(17) In caring for a patient with a vaginal discharge, the nurse must be especially careful to protect herself from possible infection by

(a) Carrying out proper handwashing techniques.
(b) Using strict isolation techniques.
(c) Giving the patient antiseptic vaginal douches.

Mr. E. had a suprapubic prostatectomy.

(18) The postoperative nursing care included all of the usual postoperative nursing duties with special emphasis on the observance for

(a) An upper respiratory infection
(b) Hemorrhage
(c) Nausea and vomiting

(19) In helping to preserve Mr. E.'s dignity, the nurse should:

(a) Request the male attendant to accompany her when changing the patient's suprapubic dressings.
(b) Explain to the patient that certain phases of his care are as embarrassing to her as they are to him.
(c) Approach him in a matter-of-fact manner.

PART VII

THE OBSTETRIC PATIENT

Chapter 44

PRENATAL CARE

REFERENCES

Bleier, I. J.: Maternity Nursing. 2nd ed. Philadelphia, W. B. Saunders Co., 1966, Chapters 1-5 and Appendix 2-4.
Culver, V.: Modern Bedside Nursing, Chapter 52.
Hoffman, C. P., Lipkin, G. B., and Thompson, E. M.: Simplified Nursing, pp. 533-548.
Rapier, D. K., et al.: Practical Nursing, pp. 449-456.
Rasmussen, S.: Foundations of Practical and Vocational Nursing, pp. 559-565.
Thompson, E. M., and Murphy, C.: Textbook of Basic Nursing, pp. 641-654.

JOURNAL

Bailey, Minnie: The unmarried pregnant teenager. Bedside Nurse, 1:13, July-Aug. 1968.

1. Color the parts of the female pelvis in Figure 56.

   A. Vertebrae - blue
   B. Colon - red
   C. Bladder - yellow
   D. Uterus and vagina - green
   E. Symphysis pubis - brown

   Conception may occur any time during 3 days as egg passes from ovary to uterus. Most fertile time is 24 hr. after ovulation.

2. In what part of the female reproductive system does the sperm meet the ovum? In the Fallopian tube

3. Describe the menstrual cycle and explain when it is possible for conception to occur. Vaginal discharge q 28 days; FSH from pituitary sends message to ovary to mature follicle + egg cell. Follicle moves to wall of ovary, breaks, then goes to uterus. If conception has not occurred lining of uterus is shed.

4. List five changes which occur in the female reproductive system as a result of pregnancy.

   1) Breasts enlarge, become tender, have a tingling sensation
   2) Uterus enlarges
   3) Vagina takes on a bluish color (congestion - Chadwick's sign)
   4) Cervix softens (Hegar's sign)
   5) Corpus Luteum enlarges + remains

5. What is the length of pregnancy in days? weeks? months?

   280 40 10 lunar
   9 calendar

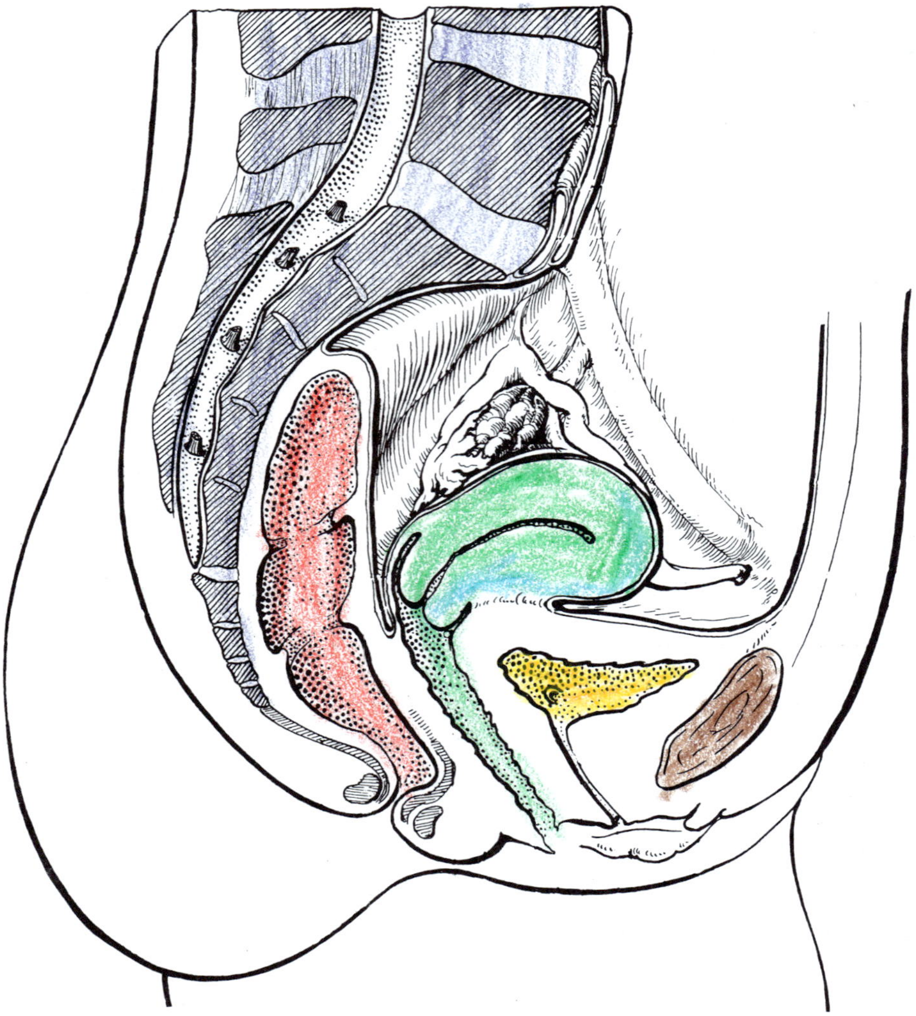

Fig. 56. Female pelvis. (Denoyer-Geppert Company, Chicago, Illinois.)

6. Complete the tables.

A. Signs of pregnancy.

PROBABLE SIGNS striae	POSITIVE SIGNS
1- Abd. changes - size - Linea Nigra 2- Reproductive organ changes - enlargement of the uterus - color change in cervix + vagina - cervix softens - Hegar's sign 3- pregnancy Tests	1- presence of fetal heart tone @ 4 1/2 months 2- fetal movement detected by a trained person 3- Visualization by xray of fetal skeleton.

Chadwick's sign

B. Tests for pregnancy.

TEST	HOW PERFORMED	PRACTICAL NURSE RESPONSIBILITIES
Ascheim–Zondek	Urine injected IM into Mouse	Collect urine early morning 3 consecutive
Friedman's	urine injected IM into Rabbit	Collect first early morning urine specimen

7. During which month in fetal development can each of the following be noted:

   A. Hearing fetal heart tones - after 4 1/2-5 months

   B. Determining the sex of the fetus - 4th month

   C. Fetal movements felt by the mother - 5th month

8. If an acquaintance of yours asked you these questions, how would you answer?

   A. "Why is it so important for me to visit a doctor for pregnancy? My mother never went to a doctor and she had five healthy children." Because many advancements have been made and the time to prevent trouble is before it starts. It is a good way to protect your health & the baby

   B. "I am three days late for my monthly period. Should I go to a doctor?" I would call the Dr. and advise him of your symptoms and let him arrange for an appointment.

   C. "This is my first pregnancy. What kind of examination will the doctor give me on my first visit to his office? Will I have the same kind of examination each time I visit him?" He will take a history the 1st time [illegible] past [illegible] menstrual periods a general exam [illegible] pelvic exam + lab tests. Next visits will be weight BP + urine check + checks for complications

   D. "What clothes shall I buy for the baby I'm expecting?" Diapers - shirts - gowns - blankets - bed - sheets - pins - sweaters

   E. "Is there anything I can do about morning sickness? How long will this sickness last?" Eat six small meals. eat before going to bed - before getting up eat dry crackers. eat dry + liquids separately. Lasts to end of 6th week

9. Name five danger signals of complications of pregnancy.

   1. Swelling of face & hands
   2. Excessive - extended nausea & vomiting
   3. headache c̄ blurred vision or spots before the eyes
   4. pain in abdomen (unusual) or cramps
   5. Bleeding from vagina or loss of fluid (uncontrollable)
   6. fever or chills

10. What should be the maximum weight gain during pregnancy?

    15-20 lbs.

11. What are the dietary needs of an expectant mother? Well balanced increase milk to 1 qt. fruits - fresh vegetables 4 or more servings - cereals & bread - 4 or more servings Meat 2 or more servings.

12. What instructions are usually given to the expectant mother in regard to

    A. Exercise? Moderate exercise. Normal activities ok. Avoid strenuous tiring exercise in last months.

    B. Care of breasts? Wear a well fitting brassiere & change size when needed. Should support breasts upward & outward. Wash breasts throughly every day. c̄ warm soapy water, rinse & dry. May apply oil, lanolin or petroleum jelly

C. Care of teeth? Good diet, cleanliness & dental check early in pregnancy.

D. Types of clothing to wear? Comfortable - not tight good bra undergarments - no garters - low well supporting shoe

E. Bathing? Frequent shower or bath to eliminate wastes. Care to be taken in lasts months to prevent falling

13. Identify and label the instruments shown in Figure 57 used in examining the obstetric patient.

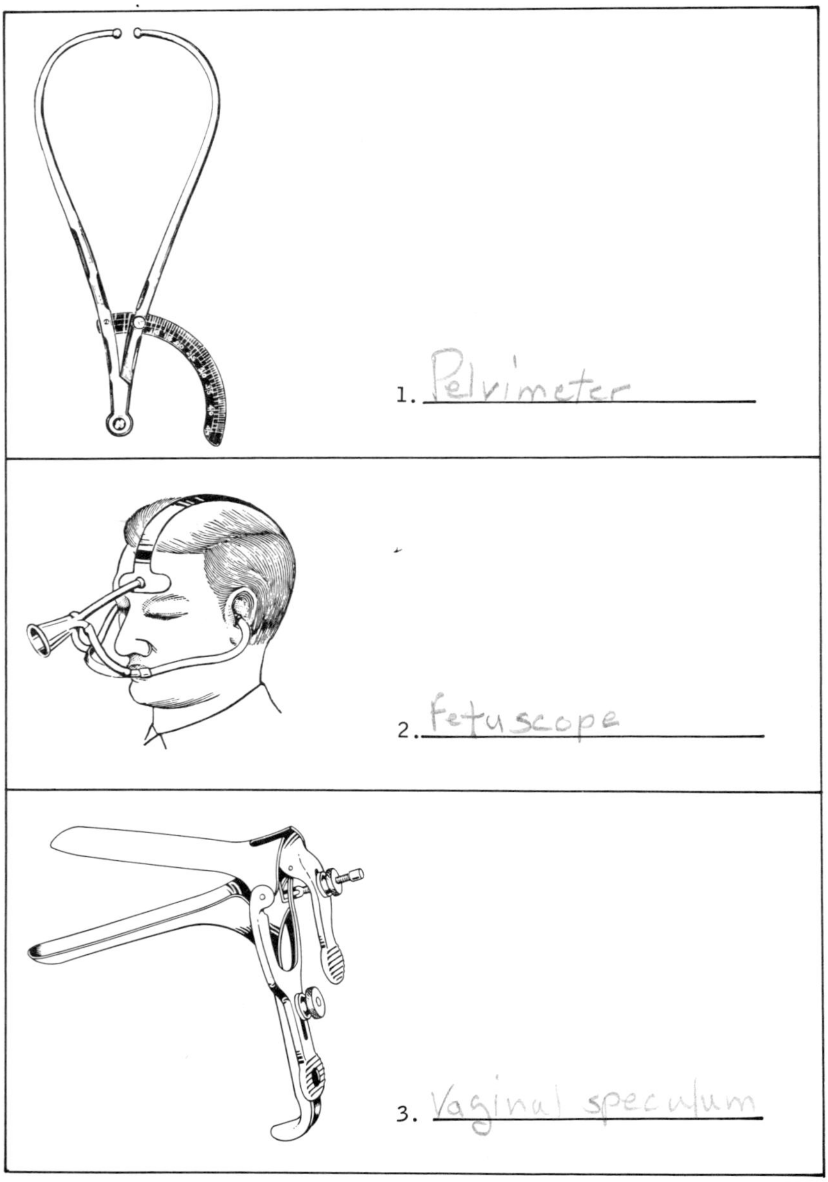

Fig. 57. Instruments used in examining the obstetric patient. (Dittmar and Penn Corporation, Philadelphia.)

14. Match each term with the correct definition.

Term		Definition
a. Trimester	c	1. The fetus drops lower into the mother's pelvis
b. Quickening	d	2. Thin watery secretion from the breasts
c. Lightening	b	3. Feeling fetal movements
d. Colostrum	e	4. Dark line extending from the pubis to the sternum
e. Linea nigra	a	5. One-third of the length of normal pregnancy

Chapter 45

LABOR AND DELIVERY

REFERENCES

Bleier, I. J.: Maternity Nursing, Chapters 7-10.
Culver, V.: Modern Bedside Nursing, Chapter 52.
Hoffman, C. P., Lipkin, G. B., and Thompson, E. M.: Simplified Nursing, pp. 551-555.
Rapier, D. K., et al.: Practical Nursing, pp. 460-461.
Rasmussen, S.: Foundations of Practical and Vocational Nursing, pp. 571-575.
Thompson, E. M., and Murphy, C.: Textbook of Basic Nursing, pp. 659-663.

JOURNAL

Cameron, Shirley: The nurse's role in the first stage of labor. J. Practical Nursing, 15:30, Jan. 1965.

---

1. Define:

   A. Labor - The process by which the products of conception are expelled

   B. Multi- More than one

   C. -gravida The number of pregnancies a woman has had.

   D. -para The number of viable pregnancies a woman has had.

   E. Prima- Primary or first.

2. List the reasons for performing each procedure during labor.

   A. Cleansing enema - To cleanse rectum so it won't contaminate - To make a wider passage. To encourage contractions

   B. Perineal "prep". To prevent infection. To make episiotomy easier. To make post partum peri care easier.

   C. Timing uterine contractions To evaluate the ability of the uterus to contract. To detect inability of the uterus to relax

   D. Checking fetal heart tones To detect fetal distress & To detect fetal life on admission. To reassure the patient

3. What is the usual duration of each stage of labor?

   A. First Primipara 8-20 hrs
   Multipara 3-8 hrs.

   B. Second Primipara 30 min to 2 hrs
   Multipara 20 min. to 1 1/2 hrs

   C. Third Primipara 5-20 min
   Multipara 5-20 min } usually aided by oxytocics

4. During which stage of labor does each of the following usually occur? Signify by placing the number 1, 2, or 3 on the line preceding the statement:

1 A. Bloody show
1 B. Uterine contractions occuring every 2 minutes and lasting 45 seconds
1 C. Rupture of membranes
2 D. Delivery of the baby
2 E. Involuntary urge to bear down
3 F. Delivery of the placenta

5. During which stage of labor is each procedure performed? Signify by placing the number 1, 2, or 3 on the line preceding the statement:

1 A. Encourage the patient to relax during and between uterine contractions.
2 B. Encourage the patient to relax between contractions and bear down during contractions.
3 C. Watch for signs of hemorrhage.
1 D. Check fetal heart tones.
2 E. Episiotomy performed when necessary.
1 F. Rectal examination.
2 G. Administration of anesthesia.
2 H. Cleanse vaginal canal with an antiseptic.
1 I. Shave perineum.
1 J. Give cleansing enema.

6. List the reason for performing each procedure immediately following the delivery

A. Check the mother's blood pressure and pulse. To detect signs of hemorrhage (low presure) To detect signs of toxemia (high pressure)

B. Massage the uterus. To keep uterus contracted + prevent hemorrhage.

C. Administer Ergotrate or similar drug. To contract the uterus + prevent hemorrhage

D. Place 1% silver nitrate drops in each of the newborn infant's eyes. To prevent a contact gonorrheal infection.

7. List five danger signals of complications which may occur during labor.
1- frank vaginal bleeding.
2- Meconium stained amniotic fluid
3- Irregular fetal heart tone
4. change in B/P
5- Prolapsed cor showing in vagina

8. How can the practical nurse help to ease the patient's fears during the labor period? By staying c̄ her and listening to her
Giving encouragement
Helping her to breath + relax

9. What type of diet is usually ordered for the patient during labor?
NPO or sips of H2O or 7up unless otherwise ordered.

10. How can the practical nurse contribute toward the practice of good medical asepsis in the labor and delivery room? By knowing what is to remain sterile - how to handle sterile supplies - proper washing - gowning and gloving technique + By reporting errors immediatly.

Chapter 46

POSTPARTUM CARE

REFERENCES

Bleier, I. J.: Maternity Nursing, Chapter 12.
Culver, V.: Modern Bedside Nursing, Chapter 52.
Hoffman, C. P., Lipkin, G. B., and Thompson, E. M.: Simplified Nursing, pp. 556-560.
Rapier, D. K., et al.: Practical Nursing, p. 462.
Thompson, E. M., and Murphy, C.: Textbook of Basic Nursing, pp. 664-668.

True or False. Circle T if the statement is true; F if the statement is false. Correct the statements that are false by crossing out the incorrect word or words and writing the correct word or words in the space above.

T F 1. The emotional feelings a mother experiences immediately following the birth of a child are usually ~~those of depression and frustration~~. They are one of elation + satisfaction

T F 2. The mother is usually given ~~nothing by mouth for at least twenty-four hours after delivery~~. her 1st meal a few hours after delivery or as ordered by Dr.

T F 3. The process of the body's returning to normal following delivery is called involution.

T F 4. The presence of bright red lochia which continues more than twelve hours after delivery should be reported immediately since this is a sign of postpartum hemorrhage.

T F 5. The breasts begin to secrete milk approximately ~~two to four hours postpartum~~. Two to four days.

T F 6. A mother may complain of abdominal cramps while breast feeding her infant because the infant's sucking stimulates uterine contractions.

T F 7. Since menstruation is usually delayed during breast feeding, the mother who breast feeds ~~cannot~~ become pregnant. Ovulation without menstruation may occur + pregnancy may result.

T F 8. ~~After-pains are usually more severe after the delivery of the first child than after the second or third child.~~ The muscle tone is poorer after the 2nd + subsequent deliveries and this makes after pains more severe.

T F 9. Perineal care is important ~~only while the mother is on bed rest.~~ during the entire period of healing to prevent infection

~~This procedure is usually discontinued when the mother becomes ambulatory.~~

T F 10. Proper support of the breasts may relieve pain associated with engorgement.

2. Match each medication with the correct action.

Medication		Action
a. Stilbestrol	e-b	1. Contracts the uterus
b. Ergot	a	2. Aids in drying up the breasts
c. Codeine	c	3. Analgesic
d. Milk of magnesia	d	4. Laxative
e. Pitocin		

3. Explain how the practical nurse can contribute toward teaching the obstetric patient in each of the following areas:

A. Personal hygiene Washing & protecting the breasts during initial breast care can be taught. Peri care: cleaning - using sprays & placing peri pad from front to back are taught before mother ambulates.

B. Healthy mother-child relationships By showing mother how to hold and feed baby - teaching that large amounts of love are given at this time. Telling her how important cuddling & loving is.

4. Multiple Choice. Circle the number preceding the correct answer to each statement.

A. Following delivery, the uterus should be

(1) Firm.
(2) Soft.
(3) Neither of these.

B. The normal discharge from the uterus following delivery is called

(1) Colostrum.
(2) Meconium.
(3) Lochia.

C. When applying an abdominal binder to the postpartum patient, begin pinning

(1) At the bottom and work up.
(2) At the center, then pin the top and bottom.
(3) At the top and work down.

D. The purpose of perineal care cannot be accomplished if the nurse

(1) Cleanses the area, wiping from the rectum upward toward the vagina.
(2) Does not wear a mask.
(3) Fails to wear sterile gloves.

E. The postpartum patient should be encouraged to void within

(1) 2 to 4 hours after delivery.
(2) 6 to 8 hours after delivery.
(3) 12 to 16 hours after delivery.

F. If the patient has difficulty in voiding, the nurse should

(1) Immediately call the doctor.
(2) Catheterize the patient.
(3) Try methods which may help the patient to void voluntarily.

G. In order to secure the maximum benefit from a breast binder, it should be applied so that the breasts are supported

(1) Upward and inward.
(2) Downward and inward.
(3) Neither of these.

H. Daily care of the nipples for the nursing mother includes

(1) Cleansing before and after each feeding.
(2) The use of a nipple shield at each feeding.
(3) Massaging well with an ointment.

I. The length of time the postpartum patient remains in bed

(1) Is 24 to 48 hours.
(2) Has lessened over a recent period of years.
(3) Is no longer important since the use of antibiotics.

J. When discharged from the hospital, the patient should be advised to

(1) Report any type of lochia to the doctor.
(2) Take sponge baths or showers instead of tub baths for several weeks.
(3) Take daily douches.

K. When breast feeding, it is important for the mother to

(1) Lie down to feed the baby.
(2) Sit up to feed the baby.
(3) Keep her breast away from the infant's nose.

L. Soreness and cracking of the nipples should be prevented since this predisposes toward

(1) Breast engorgement.
(2) Infection.
(3) A diminished secretion of milk.

M. A procedure which is given specifically to promote healing and reduce the discomfort of an episiotomy is

(1) The use of a heat lamp.
(2) Catheterizing the patient.
(3) Perineal care.

N. The postpartum period begins with the delivery of the baby and ends

(1) In six weeks.
(2) When the mother is discharged from the hospital.
(3) When the reproductive system has returned to normal.

O. For the mother who is not nursing her baby, menstruation returns in

(1) 6 to 8 weeks.
(2) 12 to 14 weeks.
(3) 16 to 20 weeks.

Chapter 47

CARE OF THE NEWBORN

REFERENCES

Bleier, I. J.: Maternity Nursing, Chapter 14.
Culver, V.: Modern Bedside Nursing, Chapter 53.
Hoffman, C. P., Lipkin, G. B., and Thompson, E. M.: Simplified Nursing, pp. 562-570.
Rapier, D. K., et al.: Practical Nursing, Chapter 49.
Rasmussen, S.: Foundations of Practical and Vocational Nursing, pp. 576-577.
Thompson, E. M., and Murphy, C.: Textbook of Basic Nursing, pp. 670-676.

JOURNALS

Appraising the newborn. J. Practical Nursing, 16:25, Sept. 1966.
Harned, Mabel: The art of modern diapering. J. Practical Nursing, 15:30, May 1965.

1. Place a check mark in front of each statement which is true concerning the characteristics of the normal newborn infant.

✓ A. The skin is covered with a cheesy material called vernix caseosa.
✓ B. The neck is short.
__ C. He sleeps about 12 hours a day.
✓ D. His eyes do not focus.
__ E. The skin is bluish in color.
✓ F. The first voiding and defecation occur within 24 hours after birth.
✓ G. He regurgitates easily.
✓ H. The respirations are irregular.
✓ I. There is a slight weight loss during the first few days after birth.
__ J. The first stool will be soft and yellow.

2. Multiple Choice. Circle the number preceding the correct answer to each statement.

You are working in the newborn nursery and are told that Baby Smith will soon be brought to your department to be properly admitted.

A. Before the baby arrives, he will have had

a. A drop of silver nitrate 1% in each eye.	1. b, c,
b. An identification bracelet attached.	2. b, c, d
c. The umbilical cord cut and clamped.	(3.) All but e
d. A physical examination by the doctor.	4. b
e. A feeding of sterile water.	5. All

B. On admission, the infant's rectal temperature is 93.8 degrees Fahrenheit.

a. You should report this to the nurse in charge.
b. This temperature is within the normal range for newborn infants.
c. It is not uncommon for an infant's temperature to drop a degree or two shortly after birth.
d. You should recheck the temperature.

1. a, d
2. b
3. a, c, d
4. All
5. None

C. To measure the length of the baby,

(1) Turn him on his side and straighten his legs, then measure along his back.
(2) Lay him on his back and measure along the front.
(3) Hold him up by the heels and let his head rest slightly on the bassinet, then measure along the back.
(4) Lay him on his abdomen and measure along his back.

D. There are several methods used in bathing a newborn infant. One is to wipe off the excess blood and allow most of the vernix caseosa to remain on the body. It is believed that the vernix caseosa

(1) Serves as a protective covering for the skin.
(2) Helps to keep the infant warm.
(3) Allows for normal perspiration.
(4) Prevents wrinkling of the skin.

E. Oil baths may be recommended in some hospitals. When giving an oil bath,

a. Vigorously rub the oil into the skin.
b. Apply the oil gently.
c. Always remove the excess oil.
d. Never apply oil to the scalp.
e. Use oil only upon the doctor's orders.

1. a, c
2. All but a
3. All but b
4. b, c
5. b, c, e

F. When weighing the infant, the order of the procedure is to

(1) Balance the scales, place a diaper over the scales and place the undressed infant on the scales.
(2) Place a diaper over the scales, lay the undressed infant on the scales, then balance the scales.
(3) Place a diaper over the scales, balance the scales, then place the undressed infant on the scales.

G. The practical nurse noted that Baby Smith weighed 7 pounds and 8 ounces. This birth weight is

(1) Average.
(2) Below average.
(3) Above average.

H. When weighing the baby on subsequent days,

(1) It is best to weigh him in the afternoon.
(2) Always weigh him at the same time daily.
(3) Weigh him before and after feedings.

I. On admission, the nurse observes the umbilical cord.

a. It is dry.
b. The clamp may be removed in a few hours.
c. It is yellow in color.
d. A small amount of blood normally oozes from the end for several hours.
e. The cord is six to eight inches long.

1. a, c, e
2. c
3. e
4. All but d
5. None

J. Baby Smith was born at 6:00 A.M. He will receive his first feeding at

(1) 10:00 A.M.
(2) 2:00 P.M.
(3) 6:00 P.M.
(4) 10:00 P.M.

K. When feeding the infant for the first time, the practical nurse will correctly

a. Hold his head slightly elevated.
b. Burp him frequently.
c. Expect him to regurgitate.
d. Encourage him to take 3 to 4 ounces.
e. Allow him 20 to 30 minutes feeding time.

1. a, b, c
2. a, b, e
3. All but e
4. All but d
5. a, b

L. The first morning after the day of birth, the practical nurse weighed Baby Smith and noted his weight was 7 pounds and 10 ounces. She may assume that

(1) This is a usual weight gain.
(2) The weight may be incorrect and should be rechecked.

M. When the infant was three days old, he was circumcised. This is a surgical procedure to correct

(1) Phimosis.
(2) Urine retention.
(3) Sterility.
(4) Hypospadias.

N. Baby Smith's formula was prepared using the terminal sterilization method. This means

a. The formula is first mixed then poured into unsterile bottles and sterilized.
b. Each ingredient is carefully measured.
c. The nurse who prepares it wears sterile gloves.
d. Each ingredient is sterilized then mixed and poured into sterile bottles.
e. Evaporated milk is used in the formula.

1. a
2. a, b, c
3. All but d
4. All but a
5. None

O. Baby Smith's mother may correctly assume that while her infant is in the hospital newborn nursery,

a. He will become "spoiled."
b. He will cry more frequently than after he goes home.
c. He will develop a mild diaper rash.
d. His environment is aseptically clean.
e. Nursing care directed toward meeting the infant's emotional needs is entirely eliminated.

1. a, d, e
2. d, e
3. All but b
4. d
5. None

Chapter 48

COMPLICATIONS

PRENATAL COMPLICATIONS: ECTOPIC PREGNANCY, TOXEMIA, HYPEREMESIS GRAVIDARIUM, INFECTIOUS DISEASES, ANTEPARTUM BLEEDING

COMPLICATIONS OF LABOR AND DELIVERY: PROLAPSED CORD, CESAREAN SECTION

COMPLICATIONS OF THE NEWBORN: ABNORMALITIES DUE TO PRENATAL FACTORS, DISTURBANCES DUE TO THE BIRTH PROCESS, CONDITIONS ARISING FROM POSTNATAL CAUSES, JAUNDICE OF THE NEWBORN

THE PREMATURE BABY

REFERENCES

Bleier, I. J.: Maternity Nursing, Chapters 6, 11, 13, 15 and 16.
Culver, V.: Modern Bedside Nursing, Chapters 52 and 53.
Hoffman, C. P., Lipkin, G. B., and Thompson, E. M.: Simplified Nursing, pp. 548-551, 555-556, 561-562, and 570-573.
Rapier, D. K., et al.: Practical Nursing, pp. 457, 461.
Rasmussen, S.: Foundations of Practical and Vocational Nursing, pp. 565-566.
Thompson, E. M., and Murphy, C.: Textbook of Basic Nursing, pp. 654, 663, 668 and 676.

JOURNALS

Apgar, Virginia: Apgar on birth defects. J. Practical Nursing, 18:20, Oct. 1968.
Hasselmeyer, Eileen G.: The infant mortality problem in the United States. J. Practical Nursing, 19:26, Jan. 1969.

PRENATAL COMPLICATIONS

1. Ectopic pregnancy is a condition in which the fertilized ovum fails to travel from the fallopian tube into the uterus. Instead, it implants itself in the walls of the tube and grows there.

A. Symptoms: Hemorrhage - pain radiating to shoulder on side pregnancy caused by pressure on diaphragm - pain in abdomen - may go into shock.

B. Treatment:

Surgical removal of pregnancy + tube + blood replacement

2. Toxemia, a term which may refer to blood poisoning, has a different meaning when applied to obstetrics. Toxemia of pregnancy is a condition of questionable cause in which a series of abnormalities occur in the pregnant woman. Years ago this condition was almost always fatal. However, since the increase in good prenatal care, symptoms of toxemia can be detected early and treated satisfactorily. What are the symptoms?

(1) Edema of the face & hands.
(2) Blurred vision c̄ spots before the eyes.
(3) Hypertension
(4) Albuminuria
(5) Headache

3. Nausea and excessive vomiting may continue beyond the first trimester of pregnancy. If so, the condition is called hyperemesis gravidarium. What effects would this condition have upon the mother?

(1) weight loss
(2) dehydration
(3) diminished urine output

4. Infectious diseases which may occur during pregnancy are syphilis, gonorrhea, tuberculosis and German measles.

A. Which tests are performed during the prenatal period to detect

(1) Syphilis? Serology blood test

(2) Gonorrhea? Vaginal secretion smear

(3) Tuberculosis? Chest X-ray

B. Why is it important to detect these diseases early in pregnancy?
to prevent damage to the fetus & protect the mothers health

C. What danger lies in the pregnant mother's having German measles?
Congenital fetal deformity

5. As you have already learned, any vaginal bleeding which occurs during an established pregnancy is abnormal and should be reported to the physician at once. The common abnormal conditions which cause antepartum bleeding are tubal pregnancy (previously discussed), abortion, placenta previa and premature separation of the placenta (sometimes called abruptio placentae).

A. Placenta previa is a condition in which the placenta attaches itself to the lower part of the wall of the uterus rather than the upper portion. During which part of the pregnancy does the bleeding from this condition occur? Why? The latter part of pregnancy because uterine contractions may loosen abnormally placed placenta

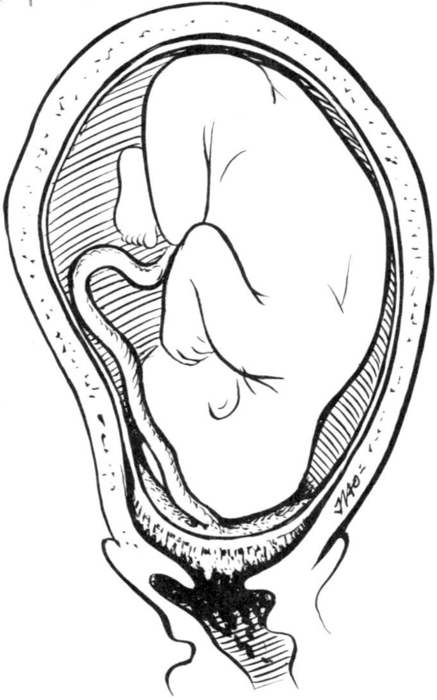

Fig. 58. Placenta previa.

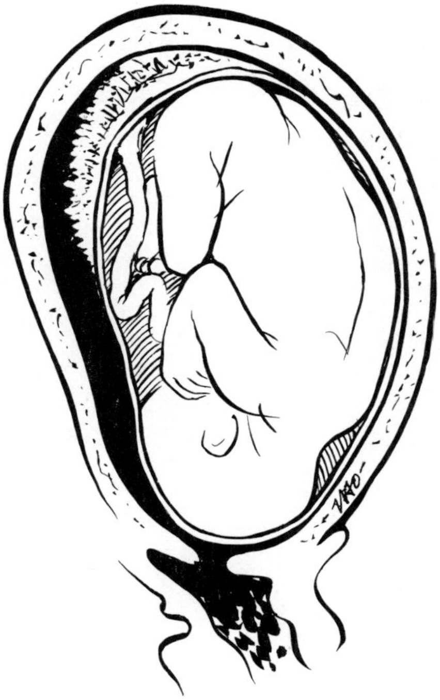

Fig. 59. Abruptio placentae. (Adapted from Bookmiller, M., and Bowen, G.: Textbook of Obstetrics and Obstetric Nursing.)

B. Abruptio placentae is a condition in which part of the placenta tears away from the walls of the uterus before the birth of the baby. See Figure 59. What are the dangers involving the

(1) Mother? May result in hidden hemorrhage + circulatory collapse + shock

(2) Baby? Loss of O_2 + nourishment to fetus

C. Abortion.

(1) Definition: Termination of a pregnancy before the 28th week may be induced or spontaneous

(2) Causes: Placenta previa - placentae abruptio - toxemia may be a defective fetus

(3) How can the practical nurse contribute to the emotional well-being of the patient who has aborted?

By reassuring her that this will in no way affect her ability to have future pregnancies + normal children. This is true in most cases + the nurse should make sure first of course - By being kind + sympathetic + understanding

COMPLICATIONS OF LABOR AND DELIVERY

1. Prolapsed cord.

   A. Definition: Cord in front of the presenting part

   B. Dangers to the infant: O_2 distress

2. Cesarean section.

   A. Give reasons for performing. Placenta Abruptio - Placenta Previa. fetal-pelvic disproportion - prolapsed cord - uterine inertia + abnormal presentations

   B. How does this type of delivery affect the appearance of the newborn? There is no molding of the head.

   C. Discuss the following concerning the postoperative nursing care of the patient who has had a cesarean section:

      (1) Is perineal care necessary? Why? yes - because of cleanliness & comfort. no heat lamps or ice because no episiotomy

      (2) How would the usual postpartum regulations for each of the following be altered?

         (a) Ambulation - may not be ordered until next day pt should be turned q2h + ambulation should be progressive

         (b) "Rooming-in"

         (c) Diet - NPO → sips of H_2O → clear liquid → soft → regular over period of 2-3 days

POSTPARTUM COMPLICATIONS

The majority of postpartum complications can be classified as infections. The infection may occur in the uterus (puerperal infection) or breasts (mastitis). Another complication is phlebitis.

1. Which disease-producing microorganisms are usually present in the lower female genital tract? Trichomonas Vaginalis & Candida albicans

2. What are the responsibilities of the nurse in preventing a puerperal infection in

   A. Prenatal period? Advising the patient to maintain good personal hygiene + report unusual symptoms stat. to the doctor

   B. Labor and delivery? Maintaining good procedures @ all times + sterile techniques when indicated.

   C. Postnatal period? Hand washing before & after caring for each pt. Proper application of peri. pads (front to back) Wiping from to back - Teaching the pt. peri care & breast care - Using only personal equipment on each pt. Using sterile drape on ice bag to protect episiotomy.

3. List the instructions which should be given to a nursing mother which would help to prevent mastitis.

1- Wash breasts first daily c̄ clea[n] wash cloth only.

2- Cover c̄ sterile beast pads.

3- Wear clean breast binder or br[a] daily.

4. Nurse for 5 min on each side at first to prevent cracks fr[om] forming which may become infected.

5- Wash hands before handling breasts when nursing.

COMPLICATIONS OF THE NEWBORN

Statistics have shown that most infant deaths occur before one month of age. Of these, one-half occur during the first twenty-four hours after birth. Thus one can see that the responsibility of the nurse in her observation of the newborn is tremendous. Since the disturbances of the newborn are too numerous to categorize in their entirety, a few will be discussed in groups according to the factors which cause them.

1. Those caused by prenatal factors. This group of conditions includes the congenital abnormalities.

A. Congenital syphilis. If a women is infected with syphilis at the time of pregnancy, the disease may be transmitted to the fetus. The fetus usually does not become infected until the fourth month of growth. If the mother begins treatment early in pregnancy, this would allow her ample time to be treated and cured before endangering her child.

(1) What is the treatment for syphilis? Antibiotic therapy

(2) How does the present incidence of congenital syphilis compare with the incidence 20 years ago? Don't know the exact rate, but the prenatal serology test has made it much less common.

B. Spina bifida. Define.
Means divided spine or a part of the posterior spine is missing. May be hidden (not serious) or may involve serious deformity c̄ protrusion of the meninges.

C. Hydrocephalus. Define.
Condition in which the cerebrospinal fluid is not reabsorbed properly in the ventricles of the brain and it accumlates in the cranium.

D. Pyloric stenosis.
Narrowing of the pyloric valve preventing passage of food.

(1) Symptoms:
occasional vomiting - becoming more frequent & forceful (projectile) dehydration malnutrition - electrolyte imbalance, weight loss.

(2) When do the symptoms first appear?
Usually at two weeks - Rarely as late as two months.

E. Harelip and cleft palate.

(1) Definition of each: Harelip is incomplete formation of the tissues of the lip on either or both sides of the upper lip. Cleft palate is lack of fusion of the hard or soft palate or the entire roof of the mouth.

(2) Treatment: Harelip is usually repaired early (2 mos) surgically. Until surgery feeding must be done carefully.
Cleft palate is usually repaired later (4 yrs) surgically and may require more than one surgery. Great care must be taken to prevent aspiration when feeding.

2. Disturbances due to the birth process. This includes such conditions as fractures and skin trauma. Which bone is fractured most frequently during the process of birth? Clavicle (collar bone)

Other abnormalities which come under this group are the disturbances of respiration. This is one of the leading causes of neonatal death. Two common abnormalities of respiration are asphyxia and atelectasis.

A. Define each. Asphyxia is lack of O_2 c̄ carbon dioxide buil
Incomplete expansion of the lungs is calle
atelectasis.

B. What standard equipment to treat asphyxia do most hospitals have in the delivery room? O_2

3. Conditions which arise from postnatal causes include infections, the most common being thrush, impetigo, epidemic diarrhea of the newborn and infections of the umbilical cord. List the procedures carried out in the newborn nursery which help to prevent these infections. Name as many as you can.

1. Good personal hygiene by nurses + all personal
2. adequate space
3. Cord care
4. No interchage of equipment or supplies between babies.
5. Use of disenfectant + technique papers on equipment used by all.
6. Use of scrub gowns + caps by personal

4. Another condition affecting infants is jaundice of the newborn, called icterus neonatorum. This condition is not serious and requires no treatment. The jaundice appears any time from the second to fifth day after birth and may last from one to several days. During this time the infant is usually listless and may be difficult to feed. Jaundice of the newborn results from the rapid destruction of the excessive red blood cells present in the newborn. If jaundice appears before the second day after birth, it must be brought to the doctor's attention as this is usually a sign that something more serious is wrong.

This might indicate the presence of erythroblastosis (RH factor) or AB-O incompatability.

THE PREMATURE INFANT

The definition of prematurity may vary in each institution. In most cases, an infant who weighs less than 2500 grams ($5\frac{1}{2}$ lb.) at birth is considered premature, regardless of the period of gestation.

Some of the more common causes of premature births include multiple births, toxemia, uterine bleeding, and acute and chronic systemic disease. Approximately 6 per cent of all live births are premature, and almost half of all the infants who die during the first postnatal month are premature.

1. What are the characteristics of the premature infant?

1. Wrinkled old man appearance (no subcutaneous fat)
2- lanugo- body hair
3- large head + abdomen
4. No molding of skull
5- irregular respirations.
6- weak or absent sucking reflex

2. What is the purpose of the incubator in the care of the premature infant?

To provide a warm sheltered environment
Can also regulate O_2 + humidity

PART VIII

THE PEDIATRIC PATIENT

Chapter 49

UNDERSTANDING THE SICK CHILD

REFERENCES

Culver, V.: Modern Bedside Nursing, Chapter 54.
Hoffman, C. P., Lipkin, G. B., and Thompson, E. M.: Simplified Nursing, pp. 577-579.
Rapier, D. K., et al.: Practical Nursing, Chapter 53.
Thompson, E. D.: Pediatrics for Practical Nurses. Philadelphia, W. B. Saunders Co., 1965, Chapter 3.
Thompson, E. M., and Murphy, C.: Textbook of Basic Nursing, pp. 681-684.

JOURNALS

Berger, Miriam K.: Family-centered nursing: rooming-in. J. Practical Nursing, 15:33, Sept. 1965.
Harwood, Dorothy: Maternal deprivation and the two-year-old. J. Practical Nursing, 18:23, April 1968.

1. True or False. Circle T if the statement is true; F if the statement is false. Correct the statements that are false by crossing out the word or words that are incorrect and writing the correct word or words in the space provided.

T F 1. Children may behave rudely because they feel insecure and neglected.

T F 2. Since children usually are terrified by the thought of hospitalization, it is best for the parents to take them to the hospital without telling them why they are going.

T F 3. Most children have very little sense of modesty.

T F 4. The pediatric nurse must be specially trained to care for children because the basic emotional needs of children are different from those of adults.

T F 5. The attitude of the nurse when admitting a child to the hospital may influence the amount of tension felt by both the child and the parents.

T F 6. Pediatric nursing procedures are the same in all hospitals.

T F 7. Children are sometimes temporarily restrained if they become violent or unmanageable.

T F 8. As a safety measure, rubber tubing should be placed on the tips of medicine droppers when used.

T F 9. The best way to put an infant's arm through a shirt sleeve is to pull it through.

T F 10. The temperature of all children under twelve years of age is taken rectally because this method is more accurate.

T F 11. Children are as capable as adults of detecting inefficiency on the part of the nurse.

T F 12. During a child's hospitalization, the nurse should not use disciplinary actions since this may add to the child's emotional tensions and fears.

T F 13. Puzzles are a suitable recreation for a six-year-old child.

T F 14. One can expect the child to be upset when the parents leave after their first few visits to the hospital.

T F 15. In order to give good nursing care in the pediatric department, the nurse should know something about the child's home life.

2. Discussion.

A. How are each of the following procedures adapted to child care?

(1) Enema.

(2) Taking the pulse rate.

(3) Oxygen therapy.

(4) Administering medications.

(5) Collection of urine specimens.

B. How would you deal with each of these situations?

(1) You observe a young graduate nurse forcing an infant to eat by holding his nose shut.

(2) You are caring for Joanne, age seven, in her home. Her brothers, ages three and four, want you to give them the same attention, types of food, etc., that you give to Joanne.

(3) Billy, age six, is in the convalescent stage of his illness but is not yet allowed out of bed. He has frequent quarrels with the other children in the ward, which usually result in his throwing all his toys and books on the floor.

Chapter 50

CHILDHOOD DISEASES

DISEASE CONDITIONS: HARELIP AND CLEFT PALATE, TONSILLECTOMY AND ADENOIDECTOMY, PYLORIC STENOSIS, UPPER RESPIRATORY INFECTIONS, OTITIS MEDIA, RHEUMATIC FEVER, CEREBRAL PALSY, ACCIDENTS, COMMUNICABLE DISEASES

GENERAL NURSING CARE

REFERENCES

Culver, V.: Modern Bedside Nursing, Chapter 53.
Hoffman, C. P., Lipkin, G. B., and Thompson, E. M.: Simplified Nursing, pp. 579-582.
Rapier, D. K., et al.: Practical Nursing, Chapters 53 and 54.
Thompson, E. M., and Murphy, C.: Textbook of Basic Nursing, pp. 684-689

JOURNAL

Bassett, Frank H.: Practical aspects of nursing the cerebral palsied child. J. Practical Nursing, 16:21, May 1966.

DISEASE CONDITIONS

1. Harelip and cleft palate. Harelip is an incomplete closure of the upper lip. Cleft palate is an incomplete closure of the roof of the mouth. Both openings are congenital and may appear on one or both sides of the mouth. The conditions very often accompany one another. The treatment for both is surgery.

A. What are the usual hospital routines for feeding an infant with these conditions May be fed c̄ rubber tipped eye dropper - Brecht feeder - asepto syringe - special nipple

(1) Preoperatively? should be fed slowly + held upright to prevent regurgitation + bubbled frequently.

(2) Postoperatively? Usually fed by gavage for the first days to 1 week. Then from clear liquid → to full liquid over a week. Rinse mouth after feeding!

B. How is the infant kept from picking or scratching at the incision?

By restraining his arms.

2. Tonsillectomy and adenoidectomy. Frequent attacks of tonsillitis, chronic infections and enlargement of the tonsils and adenoids are the leading reasons for the surgical removal of the tonsils and adenoids.

A. What are the complications of chronic tonsillitis? Chronic inflammation - recurrent pharyngitis middle ear infection

B. What is the greatest postoperative danger in a tonsillectomy?

Hemorrhage

C. Discuss the postoperative care in relation to

(1) Observance for hemorrhage. Check pulse + respirations skin color - drainage - excessive swallowing

(2) Prevention of hemorrhage. Keep patient quiet Do not allow drinking from straw. Soft bland foods No rough foods Ice collar

D. What liquids should be avoided following a tonsillectomy?

Hot liquids + tart juices

3. Pyloric stenosis is a congenital condition in which the pyloric sphincter does not open properly. The symptoms arise from the fact that one or more feedings may accumulate in the stomach.

A. At what age do the symptoms usually occur? 2 weeks. Rarely as late as 2 months.

B. List the characteristics of the vomiting.

Forceful + Frequent

C. What methods may be used to treat the condition temporarily?

Use of a heavy thickened formula and antispasmodic drugs

D. Discuss the methods of feeding the infant postoperatively.

(1) Bubble well before and after feeding.
(2) Hold baby at a steep incline (4) Place on right side after feeding.
(3) Fed small weak feedings often

4. Upper respiratory infections, which usually begin as common colds, occur frequently among preschool children.

A. In caring for a child with an upper respiratory infection in the home, what would you do if

(1) The child's temperature suddenly went to 104 degrees Fahrenheit?

Attempt to lower temp stat c̄ an alcohol rub or tepid bath - give proper dose of aspirin Call the doctor.

(2) He developed a croupy cough at 2:00 A.M.?

Place in a steamy bath room or use a vaporizer but only with proper supervision.

(3) He refused to stay in your improvised steam tent?

Take him into a steam filled bath room instead

B. Describe the action of cough medicines. They either increase or decrease mucus secretion and help loosen the mucus or lessen the urge to cough

C. What is the usual method of administering antibiotics to children?

IM

D. Plan a day's menu for a child with a sore throat.

(1) Breakfast - apple juice - soft cooked egg bowl of hot cereal
(2) Lunch - soup (vegetable) strained fruit c̄ cottage cheese - jello Milk
(3) Mashed potatoes - Meat patty - cooked carrots pudding - Milk

5. Otitis media, or middle ear infection, is a common childhood complication of upper respiratory infections. The usual treatment consists of administering antibiotics. If there is danger of the ear drum's rupturing, the doctor will surgically puncture a small opening in the ear drum. This operation is called a myringotomy and is performed because an even cut into the ear drum heals with less scar formation than does an uneven tear.

A. How does an infection spread from the throat to the middle ear?

Through the eustachian tube which shorter, broader + more horizontal in children

B. What is the average dosage of aspirin for

(1) An infant? Uder a year to be carefully calcula by Dr. usually 1/4 of a 5 gr tablet

(2) A preschool child? 1 gr (comp.) per year of age up to 5 gr not more than 6 times at 4 hr interva

C. What are the complications of otitis media?
Hearing loss. mastoiditis

6. Rheumatic fever is a disease characterized by pain in the joints and inflammation of the heart. The child may have one or many attacks of the disease.

A. Discuss the incidence of the disease.
Incidence is decreasing, but still a major cause of acquired heart disease p. 590 maternal & Chi Health - my only so

B. Name the causative organism.
Group A beta-hemolytic streptococcus.

C. What are the predisposing factors?
1 Damp climate
2 family tendency
3 Respiratory infections
4 Poor nutrition

D. Symptoms:
1 Fever & sore throat
2 Joint pain & inflammation & swelling
3 Pulse increase
4 Fatigue
5 Poor appetite
6 Bleeding tendencies

E. Treatment:
1 Bed rest
2 Antibiotics
3 Good diet

F. Describe St. Vitus' Dance. Nervous disorder c̄ muscle spasm - emotional instability and irritability - stammering - insomnia

7. Cerebral palsy, one of the leading cripplers of children, is a disturbance of voluntary muscular action due to damage of part of the brain. The extent of the disablement depends on the extent of damage in the brain.

A. How can one detect this condition? 1 Muscle spasm
2 Staggering gait 3 Indistinct halting speech - Involuntary movements

B. What are the other leading child cripplers?
Congenital heart defects - accidents

C. List some of the health agencies in your community which aid in the rehabilitation of crippled children. Casa Colina. March of Dimes - Crippled Childrens Hospital

8. Accidents hospitalize many children. Burns, injuries due to traffic mishaps, and poison taken by mouth are the leading types of accidents.

A. Review the treatment of these conditions in the unit on emergencies in your textbook.

B. Where do accidents stand among the leading causes of death in children?
Kill more children in US that the next four leading causes of death each year

9. Common communicable diseases.

A. Match each communicable disease with the correct characteristic symptom.

Communicable Disease		Characteristic Symptom
a. Whooping cough	b	1. Bluish white spots in the mouth
b. Measles	e	2. Grayish membrane covering the throat
c. Mumps	c	3. Swelling of the paratid glands
d. Chickenpox	d	4. Rash develops into blisters
e. Diphtheria	a	5. Paroxysms of coughing

GENERAL NURSING CARE

Multiple Choice. Circle the letter preceding the correct answer to each statement.

1. The term infant refers to the

   A. First six months.
   B. First year.
   C. First two years.

2. The highest rate of infant deaths occurs in the first

   A. Week.
   B. Month.
   C. Year.

3. The newborn infant usually begins to regain its weight on the

   A. First to second day.
   B. Second to fifth day.
   C. Fifth to tenth day.

4. The child should be toilet trained by the age of

   A. Two years.
   B. Three years.
   C. When he shows interest in doing so.

Douglas, age four, was brought to the hospital accident ward by his parents. He had laryngotracheitis and was admitted to the hospital.

5. The practical nurse who admitted Douglas carried out this procedure efficiently because she

   A. Loves children.
   B. Observes and tries to understand the actions and responses of the child and his parents.
   C. Thoroughly understands the disease and its symptoms, treatment and nursing care.

6. In helping Douglas adjust to the hospital, the practical nurse can help most by

   A. Reporting his symptoms to the nurse in charge.
   B. Remaining quiet and allowing Douglas to do all the talking.
   C. Explaining each procedure in detail.

7. Douglas's mother visited him the next day and handed the nurse a jar of homemade vegetable soup she had brought. The nurse's best reply would have been,

   A. "I'm sure Douglas will enjoy the soup. But first we'll have to check to see if it will be allowed on his diet."
   B. "That is very thoughtful of you. I'll give it to him for lunch today."
   C. "Visitors are not allowed to bring food of any kind into the pediatric department."

8. Douglas was placed in a croupette to relieve

   A. Tachycardia.
   B. Dyspnea.
   C. Fever.

9. A common complication of an upper respiratory infection in children is

   A. Otitis media.
   B. Pertussis.
   C. Abscessed teeth.

10. The operation performed to open the tympanic membrane is called

    A. Myringotomy.
    B. Tracheotomy.
    C. Lobotomy.

Mary, age eight, was admitted to the hospital with rheumatic fever.

11. This disease is

    A. Communicable.
    B. A crippler.
    C. Congenital.

12. Rheumatic fever usually occurs

    A. During adolescence.
    B. Following a streptococcal infection.
    C. During the summer.

13. The main objective in the treatment of Mary's condition is

    A. The relief of pain.
    B. Providing a highly nutritional diet.
    C. To prevent damage to the heart.

14. When Mary felt better, she enjoyed reading. The practical nurse helped her select the proper book by choosing

    A. A washable cover.
    B. One with eye-catching pictures.
    C. Content suitable to Mary's stage of development.

Jack attended nursery school and came in contact with another child who had the measles. Jack began developing the symptoms of measles ten days later.

15. The period between the contact and the appearance of symptoms of the disease is called

    A. Incubation.
    B. Quarantine.
    C. Immunity.

16. Jack's first symptoms were

    A. A discharge from the nose.
    B. Bluish spots in the mouth.
    C. A red rash appearing on the head.

17. Measles are transmitted by secretions from the

    A. Urinary system.
    B. Rash.
    C. Respiratory system.

18. In order to prevent complications, the nursing care for Jack includes

    A. Giving only liquids by mouth.
    B. Protecting the eyes from bright lights.
    C. Using strict isolation technique.

19. The Dick test is a susceptibility test for

    A. Diphtheria.
    B. Scarlet fever.
    C. Tuberculosis.

20. Discipline is

    A. A continual process of education.
    B. Punishment.
    C. Outmoded.

PART IX

THE MENTALLY ILL PATIENT

Chapter 51

AN INTRODUCTION TO MENTAL ILLNESS

THE MEANING OF MENTAL ILLNESS
ADMISSION TO A MENTAL HOSPITAL
GENERAL NURSE-PATIENT RELATIONSHIPS
SPECIAL THERAPIES

REFERENCES

Culver, V.: Modern Bedside Nursing, Chapter 55.
Dennis, L. B.: Psychology of Human Behavior. 3rd ed. Philadelphia, W. B. Saunders Co., 1967.
Hoffman, C. P., Lipkin, G. B., and Thompson, E. M.: Simplified Nursing, pp. 485-497.
Rapier, D. K., et al.: Practical Nursing, Chapters 60-61.
Thompson, E. M., and Murphy, C.: Textbook of Basic Nursing, pp. 577-587.

---

1. Explain in your own words what you think mental illness is.

2. How have the attitudes toward mental illness changed during the past century?

3. Do you feel that the majority of the public now understands the term "mental illness?" Why?

4. What are the basic characteristics of the following mental disorders?

A. Psychoneuroses

B. Psychoses

5. What are your feelings about these statements?

A. "They say he is mentally ill, but I don't believe it. I've known him for years, and he is an intelligent man. There is nothing wrong with his brain."

B. "The only thing wrong with him is that he is full of the devil. He needs a good dose of religion."

C. "She has been going to a psychiatrist for years, and if you ask me, it's all just a money racket."

6. What are the objectives of each of the following in the approach to the problem of mental illness?

A. Mental health programs

B. Hospitalization

C. Rehabilitation

The nurse's approach to the patient who is mentally ill depends a great deal on her own understanding of and attitude toward mental illness. In the preceding discussions you have had an opportunity to evaluate your attitudes toward mental illness. The nurse's personality is another important aspect of nurse-patient relationships, since the mentally ill person is affected by the emotional responses of others.

7. In your opinion, which three personality characteristics are the most important for those dealing with emotionally disturbed persons? Why?

8. List several important observations which must be made concerning the following in the care of the mentally ill:

A. Conduct

B. Emotional reactions

C. Appetite

D. Speech

E. Sleep

9. What is meant by "specialing" a patient?

10. In addition to observations, what are the objectives of nursing care for the mentally ill?

11. In what way are each of the following useful in the treatment of the mentally ill?

A. Occupational therapy

B. Recreational therapy

C. Hydrotherapy

D. Shock therapy

E. Psychotherapy

Chapter 52

CARING FOR SPECIFIC BEHAVIOR GROUPS

SPECIFIC BEHAVIOR GROUPS: THE OVERACTIVE PATIENT, THE UNDERACTIVE PATIENT, THE OLDER PATIENT, THE CONVALESCENT PATIENT
GENERAL NURSING CARE

REFERENCES

Brown, M. M., and Fowler, G. R.: Psychodynamic Nursing. 3rd ed. Philadelphia, W. B. Saunders Co., 1966, Part III.
Culver, V.: Modern Bedside Nursing, Chapter 56.
Hoffman, C. P., Lipkin, G. B., and Thompson, E. M.: Simplified Nursing, pp. 497-508.
Rapier, D. K., et al.: Practical Nursing, Chapters 62-65.
Thompson, E. M., and Murphy, C.: Textbook of Basic Nursing, pp. 587-597.

JOURNALS

DeSalvatore, Theresa: Nursing care of the alcoholic. J. Practical Nursing, 17:31, April 1967.
Fox, Ruth: The nurse and the alcoholic. J. Practical Nursing, 16:24, Jan. 1966.

SPECIFIC BEHAVIOR GROUPS

1. The overactive patient is, as the term implies, one who shows increased mental and physical activity in varying degrees.

A. What is the usual behavior of the overactive patient?

B. What does the nursing care of the overactive patient consist of in the following areas:

(1) Nourishment

(2) Protection of patient

(3) Psychological approach to patient

2. The underactive patient is one who portrays decreased mental and physical activity in varying degrees. These patients usually feel rejected and worthless.

A. What is the usual behavior of the underactive patient?

B. What nursing procedures are carried out to attend to the underactive patient's physical needs?

3. The older patient is, of course, subject to any type of psychiatric disorder. One common disorder of the aged is called senile psychosis. This disorder is characterized by forgetfulness, disorganization of speech, disorientation to time and place, irritability and physical feebleness.

A. How can the nurse help protect the senile patient against injury?

B. How can the nurse provide activity for the senile patient?

4. The convalescent patient needs just as much care and attention as the acutely ill patient.

A. Around what objective is the care of the convalescent patient centered?

B. What special privileges may be given to the hospitalized convalescent patient?

GENERAL NURSING CARE

Multiple Choice. Circle the letter preceding the statement that is correct.

1. The following statement is true concerning mental illness.

   A. The incidence of mental illness is decreasing.
   B. All mental diseases are now curable.
   C. Mental illness is the leading health problem in the United States.
   D. All mentally ill patients are potentially dangerous to others.

2. The term insane refers to

   A. All mentally ill persons.
   B. The legal term for persons unsound of mind.
   C. Those mentally ill persons who are hospitalized.

3. The care of the mentally ill patient is centered around his

   A. Behavior.
   B. Physical needs.
   C. Need for protection.

Mary, age 32, was admitted to a psychiatric hospital. Several months prior to her admission, she had become irritable with others and seemed to have lost interest in performing her household duties. She always felt tired but had difficulty sleeping. Her appetite decreased, and she lost weight. She seemed incapable of making even the smallest decision, such as which dress to wear to a social function. When her husband mentioned her behavior to her, she became very upset and said, "I wish I were dead. That would solve everything." Her husband finally insisted that she see a doctor. The doctor suggested that Mary be admitted to a mental hospital for observation and treatment. Mary agreed that this seemed to be a worthwhile suggestion, and an admission was arranged.

4. Mary's hospital admission was a

   A. Voluntary admission.
   B. Commitment.

5. Mary's behavior may be classified as

   A. Overactive.
   B. Underactive.
   C. Senile.

6. An ever-present danger with this type patient is that of

   A. Physical injury to others.
   B. Lack of tidyness.
   C. Suicidal attempts.

7. During the first few days in the hospital, Mary talked very little to anyone. The practical nurse noticed Mary sitting in a corner of the lounge by herself, doing nothing. In attempting to start a conversation with Mary, the nurse should

   A. Approach her and say, "Why are you looking so blue? Cheer up; things could be worse!"
   B. Get a magazine and sit next to her. Find an article or picture of interest in the magazine and start a discussion about it.
   C. Leave Mary alone for the time being because she obviously doesn't want to be disturbed.

8. In attempting to get Mary to engage in diversional activity, the nurse would try to interest Mary in

   A. Helping to arrange flowers.
   B. Playing chess.
   C. Writing a poem.

9. Mary eats very little at mealtime. The nurse should

   A. Explain to her that she is losing weight and will become seriously ill if she doesn't eat.
   B. Ignore the fact, since she is only doing this to get attention.
   C. Offer her a particular food and suggest that she try it.

10. Quite unexpectedly one day, Mary seemed much more cheerful. The nurse can assume that this suddenly elated mood

    A. Is a definite sign that Mary is on the road to recovery.
    B. Could be a danger signal.
    C. Is a sign that her condition is becoming worse.

11. Matches, glassware and all sharp objects such as scissors, needles and sharp instruments are kept away from mentally ill patients. When Mary asked the nurse for a scissors to cut a dangling thread from her dress, the nurse replied,

    A. "No one is allowed to have scissors in this hospital."
    B. "I can take care of that," then proceeded to get a scissors and cut the thread herself.
    C. "It won't be necessary to remove the thread. No one will notice it."

12. While she was walking through the ward, the nurse was approached by another patient who said, "There are pixies standing on that window sill." The nurse should reply

    A. "I don't see anything on the window sill."
    B. "Yes, I see them too."
    C. "You know perfectly well there is no such thing as a pixie."

13. The most important aspect of caring for the mentally ill patient is to

    A. Help to keep him in contact with his surroundings.
    B. Help him to realize that he is behaving foolishly.
    C. Keep him from facing problems.

14. The prime function of the National Institute of Mental Health is to

    A. Prevent mental illness.
    B. Provide care for the mentally ill.
    C. Provide homes for the mentally retarded.

15. The practical nurse's best contribution toward mental illness is to

    A. Take a postgraduate course in psychiatric nursing.
    B. Help with fund-raising campaigns in her community.
    C. Realize that the mentally ill are people who have emotional problems and need help.

PART X

A STEP FORWARD

Chapter 53

YOU AND THE FUTURE

STATE BOARD EXAMINATIONS
FINDING A JOB
KEEPING UP-TO-DATE

REFERENCES

Bush, C. H.: Personal and Vocational Relationships for Practical Nurses, Chapter 12.
Chapman, A.: Opportunities in Practical Nursing. Practical Nursing 5:8, April 1955.
Practical Nurses in Civil Service. Practical Nursing 5:13, September 1955.
Rapier, D. K., et al.: Practical Nursing, Chapter 70.
Ross, C. F.: Personal and Vocational Relationships in Practical Nursing, Chapter 9.
Stevens, M. K.: Personal and Vocational Relationships of the Practical Nurse, Chapters 9 and 24.
Sutherland, J. E.: A Placement Service for Practical Nurses. Practical Nursing 6:10, May 1956.
Thompson, E. M., and Murphy, C.: Textbook of Basic Nursing, Chapter 53.
Torrap, H.: American Occupations, No. 6, Trained Practical Nurse. Boston, Research Publishing Co.

Congratulations! You have now completed your practical nursing course and are ready to make some definite decisions concerning the future. Your two main interests now are (1) passing state boards and (2) getting your first pay check. This chapter is designed to help you pursue both interests.

GOOD LUCK!

STATE BOARD EXAMINATIONS

Although the thought of state board examinations causes some anxiety for everyone, there is no need to panic. If you have done well in your work in this workbook, chances are that you will have no difficulty in passing state board examinations. To review for the examinations, study

1. The completed pages in this workbook.
2. Notes taken in class.
3. Returned tests.
4. Your practical nursing textbook.

If you feel that you want additional review, there are books designed for that purpose. Ask your instructor to recommend a suitable review book. Write the title of the book (or books) here:

1. When and where are state board examinations given in your state?

2. If you decide to move to another state, how will you obtain a license to practice in that state?

FINDING A JOB

You have undoubtedly already given considerable thought to the type of position you want. If you are undecided, ask your instructor for advice.

1. What positions are available to practical nurses in your community?

2. Which of these positions would you be most interested in? Why?

Some of the things you will be doing in applying for a job include writing a letter of application, writing a résumé, filling out an application and appearing for a personal interview.

3. Select a position you are interested in and write a letter of application.

4. Sometimes an advertisement in the newspaper or a letter from a prospective employer will request a résumé. What information should be included in a résumé?

5. What are some important points to remember in filling out an application?

6. You have sent your application for a position and have received an appointment for a personal interview. What will you wear when you go for the interview?

7. What information will you want to know about the job before you accept it?

8. If you should decide to resign from a position, how will you do it?

KEEPING UP-TO-DATE

Every nurse who wants to continue being a nurse has certain obligations to herself, to her employers and to her patient. One of these obligations is to keep abreast with what is going on in her profession. It is a mistake to think that once you have graduated, there is nothing more you can learn about nursing.

1. How can the practical nurse keep informed about changes in medical care and treatment?

2. How can the practical nurse keep informed about what is being accomplished by other practical nurses in her community, state and country?

3. What postgraduate courses are available for practical nurses in your community?

NOTES

NOTES

NOTES

NOTES

NOTES

NOTES

NOTES

NOTES

NOTES

NOTES

NOTES

NOTES